Gait Disorders

THE MOST COMMON COMPLAINTS SERIES

Headache
Egilius L. H. Spierings

Confusion
Karl E. Misulis and Terri Edwards-Lee

Neck Complaints
Michael Ronthal

Chest Pain
Richard C. Becker

Gait Disorders

Michael Ronthal, MBBCh, FRCP, FRCPE, FCP(SA)

*Associate Professor of Neurology, Harvard Medical School,
Boston; Deputy Chief of Neurology, Department of Neurology,
Beth Israel Deaconess Medical Center, Boston*

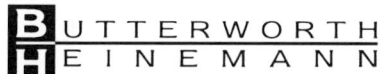

Boston   Oxford   Aukland   Johannesburg   Melbourne   New Delhi

Library of Congress Cataloging-in-Publication Data

Ronthal, Michael, 1938–
    Gait disorders / Michael Ronthal.
        p. ; cm. — (The most common complaints series)
    Includes bibliographical references and index.
    ISBN 0-7506-7337-0 (pbk. : alk. paper)
    1. Gait disorders. I. Title. II. Series.
    [DNLM: 1. Gait Ataxia—diagnosis—Aged. 2. Gait—physiology. 3. Gait Apraxia—diagnosis—Aged. WE 103 R774g 2002]
    RC376.5 .R664 2002
    616.7—dc21

                                                                    2001052782

British Library Cataloguing-in-Publication Data
A catalogue record for this book is available from the British Library.

The publisher offers special discounts on bulk orders of this book.
For information, please contact:

Manager of Special Sales
Butterworth–Heinemann
225 Wildwood Avenue
Woburn, MA 01801-2041
Tel: 781-904-2500
Fax: 781-904-2620

For information on all Butterworth–Heinemann publications available, contact our World Wide Web home page at: http://www.bh.com

10 9 8 7 6 5 4 3 2 1

Printed in the United States of America

*This book is dedicated to the memory of Norman Geschwind,
who first set me on this course, and to my wife, Berenice,
without whose encouragement and support these pages would
have forever remained "something to do one day."*

Contents

Preface

In the early 1980s, the late Norman Geschwind suggested that Lew Sudarsky and I study the problem of gait disorders in the elderly. This resulted in our initial survey of the first 50 patients presenting to our offices with the complaint, "Doctor, I can't walk." Despite technological advances over the years, I remain convinced that the diagnosis in these patients depends on a meticulous clinical examination, and as the chapters in this book were written, it dawned on me that I was producing to some extent a sophisticated, but nevertheless basic, primer in the "art" of the bedside examination.

As technology advances and becomes universally available, there is a temptation to "do the tests" at the expense of the examination. The situation is aggravated by the social changes in health care delivery that demand the clinician "process" more patients per unit time just to pay the expenses of practice. Unless we spend more time on examining the patient and individually choosing the imaging study, a decision based on the physical signs, health care costs will continue to escalate needlessly. Too often the patient comes into my office with a clutch of magnetic resonance imaging (MRI) scans; every one is an image of a part of the nervous system irrelevant to the clinical localization and every one drives up the cost of medical care. It has been said that a good neurologic consultation is by far cheaper than multiple MRIs of the neuraxis!

If this book reminds us that the basis of clinical neurology is still, and will forever remain, a finehoned and reproducible history and examination, it will have provided an invaluable service, quite apart from providing a modus vivendi for the diagnosis of gait disorders in the elderly.

M.R.

Introduction

Walking is easy. We do it all the time and don't think about it. Yet, when the mechanism for normal walking breaks down, the consequences can be disastrous.

It is estimated that about 15% of individuals over the age of 60 have some degree of difficulty with gait and 20–25% of people over the age of 80 use mechanical aids for walking. In one series of 100 admissions to a geriatric unit, 22 patients had gait disorders.

The purpose of this book is to provide an approach to the diagnosis of gait disorders in the office or at the bedside. An understanding of the basic pathophysiology of gait facilitates an approach to diagnosis of the cause of a gait disorder, and while some "science" inevitably creeps in, this book is more about the "art" of diagnosis. It should be possible after examination to pinpoint the basic mechanism(s) underlying the disability in almost all patients presenting with the complaint, "Doctor, I can't walk," so that investigation can be tailored to further explore the pathology.

A hands-on clinical examination is crucial to the diagnosis. Computerized gait analysis is a great academic tool but does not help the clinician faced with the diagnostic problem of a gait disorder. Therefore, in keeping with the objectives of the book, I have deliberately omitted a chapter on the subject.

How then to make a diagnosis?

The elderly patient with a gait disorder almost never comes up with a valid explanation for the deficit, and this is the one presentation in clinical neurology where a superb history is unlikely to make a diagnosis. Nevertheless, it's worth asking about cognitive symptoms and bladder function as well as obtaining general medical history.

In many ways, the examination can be likened to a detective story. One starts with a list of suspects and eliminates them one by one, being left at the end with the most likely cause. The trick is to consider the problem in terms of the most basic deficits rather than speculating about complex pathology.

At a basic level then, the neurologic examination is designed to ferret out physical signs that explain the gait disorder. Therefore, the mental status examination may target frontal lobe dysfunction, and the elementary examination is for documentation of spasticity, weakness, loss of position sense, ataxia, vestibular dysfunction, or extrapyramidal signs. At the same time, the general medical examination screens for nonneurologic causes of gait disorder. Last, if the gait disorder seems more than can be explained by the examination, the possibility of a psychogenic cause should be explored. Not infrequently, multiple abnormalities will be found in the same patient and some at least will be amenable to treatment.

The various chapters deal with each possible cause in detail, discussing basic mechanisms and describing the physical signs.

In 1983, along with Lewis Sudarsky, I surveyed patients referred because of abnormal gait and Sudarsky added another 70 patients to the initial cohort of 50 subjects. The spread of diagnoses is detailed in Table I-1. It should be noted that, in about 14% of elderly patients presenting with a gait disorder, despite an excellent examination and sophisticated investigations, the cause remains unknown.

Once the system deficit is documented at the bedside, further investigation is designed to explore the possible causes of that deficit with a view to a

Table I-1. Gait disorders in 120 patients

Etiology	Total	Percentage
Sensory deficits	22	18.3
Myelopathy	20	16.7
Multiple infarcts	18	15
Unknown cause	17	14.2
Parkinsonism	14	11.7
Cerebellar degeneration	8	6.7
Hydrocephalus	8	6.7
Other	6	5
Psychogenic	4	3.3
Toxic/metabolic	3	2.5

therapeutic intervention. About one in four patients will be found to have a treatable disorder; whether the treatment is drug based, requires physical therapy, or even requires surgical intervention, depends on the pathology.

SUGGESTED READING

Elble RJ. Clinical and research methodology for the study of gait. In JC Masdeu, L Sudarsky, L Wolfson (eds), Gait Disorders of Aging. Philadelphia/New York: Lippincott Raven, 1997.

Elble RJ, Hughes L, Higgins C. The syndrome of senile gait. J Neurol 1992;239:71.

Fife TD, Baloh RW. Disequilibrium of unknown cause in older people. Ann Neurol 1993;34:694.

Newman G, Dovermuehle RH, Busse EW. Alterations in neurologic status with age. J Am Geriatr Soc 1960; 8:915.

Prakash C, Stern G. Neurological signs in the elderly. Age Ageing 1973;2:24.

Sudarsky L, Ronthal M. Gait disorders among elderly patients: A survey of 50 patients. Arch Neurol 1983; 40:740.

Gait Disorders

The Physiology of Gait

Walking is easy. We do it all the time, usually at a subconscious level, yet the physiology is complex and sometimes difficult to understand.

Grillner, one of the pioneers in gait research suggests that three distinct types of control systems are involved. The motor system produces propulsive movements, the postural motor system maintains appropriate body orientation during ongoing locomotion, and goal-directed aspects of locomotor behavior bring the organism to the goal of the locomotor episode while avoiding objects that may impede locomotion (Table 1-1).

Much of the experimental evidence for gait initiation and control is related to ablation procedures in the cat.

Table 1-1. Physiology of gait

Motor System: Propulsive movement is generated at the
    Spinal level: *Central spinal pattern generator (CPG)*
    Brain stem level:
        Decorticate cat preparation *(Animal runs and walks
            without assistance)*
        Premamillary preparation *(Walks in response to a
            moving treadmill)*
        Postmamillary preparation *(Requires electrical or
            chemical stimulation of the mesencephalic loco-
            motor region to generate stepping)*
        Decerebrate cat preparation *(Decerebrate rigidity—
            no walking)*
        While the cerebellum modulates adjustment and
            timing of movement

Postural System: The center of gravity must be maintained over the base of support
    Input:
        Vision
        Vestibular
        Somatosensory
    Output:
        Spinal cord reflexes
        Brain stem reflexes
        Voluntary response

Goal-Directed System: Must reach the goal and avoid
impeding objects

PROPULSIVE MOVEMENT

Spinal Level

Newborn infants exhibit automatic stepping and placing movements. Even anencephalic infants will walk automatically if the feet are stimulated and the body supported; a lower level gait generator must be present. Experimental support for a central spinal pattern generator (CPG) is provided by the decerebrate and spinal cat preparations, as well as other animal models. If the lower thoracic spinal cord is transected, the spinal cat will walk on a moving treadmill with a near normal stepping pattern, given external support for balance. There is a rhythmic alteration between flexor and extensor muscles and the step cycle can be analyzed in terms of two phases—the swing phase when the foot is off the ground and the stance phase when the foot is planted and the leg extended. The spinal cat will adapt to the belt speed and change from the alternating gait of walk and trot to the in-phase pattern of gallop.

The adaptation to the speed of the treadmill belt requires sensory input to the spinal circuits coordinating locomotion. Afferents influenced by hip position affect the duration of the support phase and, in turn, influence the initiation of the swing phase when the limb is extended. Afferents influenced by the load on the muscles activated during the support phase play a prominent role in determining when the swing phase can be initiated. There are independent pattern generators for each limb.

Load receptors can be divided into

True load receptors—the Golgi tendon organ.
Body support receptors—cutaneous receptors on the sole of the feet.
Neuromuscular receptors—the muscle spindles.
Joint receptors—the Ruffini endings and Pacinian corpuscles.

Feedback information from muscles, joints, and associated tissues via proprioceptive reflex systems is required to adjust the motor program to irregularities of the ground during walking or to respond if the leg encounters resistance. Spinal reflex responses are not stereotyped to a given sensory input but, depending on the descending and segmental conditions, different available pathways are utilized, including both monosynaptic and polysynaptic reflexes.

Graham-Brown suggested that the CPG for any limb is divided into two halves, one half for extensors and one half for flexors. Interneurons controlling flexor and extensor motor neurons have reciprocal inhibitory connections; thus, if flexor neurons fire, extensor neurons are inhibited. The inhibition of extensor interneurons decreases with time because of the intrinsic limit to the duration of inhibition, and the extensor interneurons become sufficiently depolarized to fire and in turn inhibit flexor neurons, creating a cycle.

CPG networks controlling rhythmic hindlimb movements in vertebrates are distributed throughout the hindlimb enlargement of the cord and most probably also in the lower thoracic cord. This distributed nature of the network supports the notion that the CPG controlling hindlimb movements is not a unitary entity but can be subdivided into unit burst generators controlling single muscles or joints. The exact localization of the CPG in the transverse plane remains undecided, but rhythmically active neurons that respond to stimuli delivered to the locomotor producing regions of the brain stem are located in laminae VII, VIII and around the central canal.

Brain Stem Level

While the CPG can produce basic locomotor rhythm, brain stem structures are necessary to activate and regulate the rhythm in the intact and decerebrate animal. If a region contains neurons that, when activated chemically or electrically, lead to the production of locomotion, that area is classified as being a "loco-motor region." Locomotor regions within the brain stem encompass nuclei that are responsible for the control of many other diverse processes as well as locomotion.

Spinal cats that have been deafferented can still be made to walk on the treadmill by the intravenous administration of L-dopa, which stimulates mono-aminergic descending pathways from the brain stem that have not yet had time to degenerate.

Stimulation of the brain stem in the decerebrate cat can also evoke locomotion. Different types of loco-moting decerebrate cats can be prepared, depending on the level of transection of the neuraxis.

Decortication implies removal of the cortex with no particular damage to the thalamus or basal ganglia. The movements of these preparations are nearly normal, and the cats can run and walk with-out any external assistance.

In the *premamillary* preparation, transection is made immediately rostral to the superior colliculus and continued rostroventrally to the rostral tip of the mamillary bodies. These animals can walk spon-taneously in response to a moving treadmill and show righting reflexes.

The *postmamillary* preparation is made by making a cut rostral to the superior colliculi and continuing rostroventrally to a point caudal to the mamillary bodies. These cats rarely walk spontaneously and usually require either electrical or chemical stimulation of the mesencephalic locomotor region (MLR) of the brain stem to generate stepping movements.

If the transection of the neuraxis is made between the two colliculi, the *classic decerebrate* preparation of Sherrington is produced. Here, there is a high level of extensor tone, decerebrate rigidity, and the animals do not walk.

The MLR projects to the medial medullary reticular formation (MRF) and then on to interneurons in the spinal cord.

The medial MLR (mMLR) projects to the pontomedullary locomotor strip (PLS) and to the MLR to become part of the sensory activating system traveling along the dorso lateral funiculis (DLF).

Stimulation of the PLS and MRF can evoke bouts of locomotion, which tend to be a little uncoordinated and at times spastic.

The MRF and MLR received inputs from forebrain regions that lead to the production of complex locomotor behaviors. Therefore, there is a projection from hippocampus and amygdala to the nucleus accumbens and forward to the subpallidal region and the MLR. Inputs from basal ganglia and the lateral hypothalamic area likewise connect with the MLR.

To add to the complexity, other brain stem descending pathways modulate the amplitude of muscle activity in a phase-dependent manner during walking (vestibulospinal, reticulospinal, and rubrospinal tracts). Furthermore, electrical stimulation of locus ceruleus, raphe nuclei, and the cuneiform nucleus modulate electrical activity in muscles. Thus, descending brain stem pathways not only provide the tonic descending drive necessary to activate the locomotor pattern generator but also optimize reflex pathways.

The locomotor regions in the brain stem can be experimentally activated by electrical as well as by chemical stimulation. The MLR is activated by picrotoxin, bicuculline, NMDA, substance P, and glutamic acid. It can be inhibited by GABA and muscimol. The MRF is activated by glutamic acid and picrotoxin; and the PLS can be activated by glutamic acid, picrotoxin, and substance P and inhibited by GABA and muscimol.

The Cerebellar Level

During locomotion the cerebellum contributes to the adjustment of the timing of limb movement. This includes interlimb coordination during locomotion and modification of various reflex activities so that the movement matches the environmental needs. Cerebellar contribution to gait control can be achieved via presetting and adjustment of the gain of proprioceptive reflexes and also by the sequencing of programmed responses. It has also been suggested that the cerebellum has a stabilizing effect on the stretch reflex. The midline cerebellum tunes the magnitude of somatosensory loops involved in the maintenance of stance posture by adjusting the threshold or bias, but not the slope, of automatic postural responses.

The Purkinje cells are the output neurons of the cerebellar cortex and inhibit the deep cerebellar nuclei (fastigial and interpositus). During locomotion, the discharge of most Purkinje cells is modulated in the rhythm of stepping, and they discharge in bursts separated by periods of silence. The overall activity of the entire population Purkinje cells in the anterior lobe is maximal at the beginning of the stance phase, and the fastigial nucleus is maximally active in the swing phase of the ipsilateral hindlimb. The nucleus interpositus discharges maximally at the beginning of the swing phase and least in the stance phase of the ipsilateral hindlimb.

Rhythmic modulation of the rubrospinal, reticulospinal, and vestibulospinal neurons is mostly abolished after cerebellar ablation, so that it is concluded that rhythmic signals reaching the cerebellum via the spinocerebellar pathways modulate activity of the cerebellar neurons, whose output, in turn, rhythmically entrains activity of cells of origin of the descending brain stem pathways.

During locomotion, the rubrospinal, reticulospinal, and vestibular spinal nuclei show rhythmical bursting discharges. The rubrospinal neurons are excitatory to flexor motor neurons innervating the contralateral hindlimb muscles, the reticulospinal cells are excitatory and inhibitory to flexor and extensor motor neurons of the ipsilateral hindlimb and maximally active in the flexor or swing phase, while the vestibular spinal cells are excitatory to extensor alpha-motor neurons of the ipsilateral hindlimb and maximally active at the beginning of the extensor or stance phase of locomotion.

After cerebellectomy, the background activity of the vestibulospinal neurons increases and activity of the rubrospinal and reticulospinal neurons decreases. It has therefore been suggested that uncoupling of the descending pathways results in abnormal relations between flexor and extensor muscle tone causing *ataxia*.

In the decerebrate cat, stimulation of a restricted region along the midline cerebellar white matter evokes generalized augmentation of muscle tone on a stationary surface and locomotion on a treadmill.

The Vestibulospinal System Level

The cat on a treadmill preparation can be made to change gait from a slow walk to a fast walk, a trot, and even a gallop. When the gait changes from a slow walk to fast walk, recording electrodes show that vestibulospinal neurons that show single bursting discharges in the extensor phase of the ipsilateral hindlimb, exhibit double bursting discharges in a single-step cycle. Previously silent vestibulospinal neurons start to discharge tonically with a gradual increase in discharge frequency, some of them rhythmically. Single vestibulospinal neurons become capable of controlling movements of not only the ipsilateral but also the contralateral hindlimb; and ultimately, during a gallop when the hindlimbs move in phase, each of the double bursting discharges of the single vestibulospinal neurons fuse, increasing dramatically their average firing frequency. This change in the magnitude of populational activity of vestibulospinal neurons depending on internal and external demands contributes to the simultaneous control of rhythm, power, and the phase of required locomotor movements. It is likely the descending signals carried by the reticulospinal and rubrospinal pathways are also modified sequentially in this manner.

BALANCE AND POSTURE

In humans, walking and standing depend on the ability to keep the center of gravity (COG) within the vertical projections of a narrow base. Bipedal human gait consists of two single-limb relatively long support periods that together take up 75–80% of the whole gait cycle duration. During these two periods, the vertical projection of the COG travels forward and outside the medial border of the supporting foot, creating potential mediolateral instability during single-limb support periods—the body tends to fall toward the midline. Furthermore, in humans, two thirds of the total body weight is centered in the upper body, which makes for inherent instability.

Provided the COG is maintained over the base of support, the stabilizing influence of gravity is overcome and walking, reaching, or rising from a chair become possible without falling. If the COG deviates from the base of support, without a stabilizing rapid corrective step or external support, a fall would ensue.

The limits of stability have been defined as an inverted cone, with the apex at the feet, and the base defining a perimeter at the head. Sway outside of the perimeter results in instability. The dimensions of the base of the cone are roughly 12.5° in the anteroposterior (AP) diameter and 16° laterally.

To avoid a fall while standing or walking, compensatory movement strategies are used, but there is no single movement strategy for balance under all conditions. Rotating the body as an approximately rigid mass about the ankle joints is referred to as the *ankle strategy*. A rapid trunk movement about the hip joints with smaller opposing rotation to the ankle joints is called the *hip strategy*.

The position of the COG relative to the base of support must be continually monitored so that sensory feedback enables corrective action. The major sensory pathways include vision, vestibular, and somatosensory inputs. The dorsal column, medial leminiscus system conveys proprioception and tactile sensation from the contralateral body. The anterolateral system (spinothalamic, spinoreticular, and spinotectal tracts) conveys nociceptive and tactile information.

No single receptor combination for normal balance can be defined, and at times conflicting information from one source must be suppressed to avoid surface or surround movement illusions. This sorting out process has been called *sensory organization*.

The motor output responses to movement of the COG outside of the normal perimeter encompass

1. Local spinal cord reflexes triggered by myotactic stretch receptors localized to the point of

stimulus, are highly stereotyped, and have an onset time of 35–40 msecs.

2. Automatic brain stem and subcortical reflexes coordinated among the leg and trunk muscles, stereotyped but adaptable, and coordinate movements across joints. Onset time is 85–95 msecs.

3. Voluntary responses that generate purposeful behaviors and have longer onset time latencies of 150+ msecs, sometimes called *proactive balance control systems.* Vision and attention are the keys to the early detection of potential balance threats.

GOAL-DIRECTED LOCOMOTION

Sinnamon suggested that specific subsets of locomotor nuclei are associated with initiation of locomotion in different behavioral circumstances. The behavioral context of locomotion may be considered as exploratory, appetitive, and defensive. Exploratory function is part of the basal ganglia circuits, the lateral hypothalamic locomotor region is concerned with the primary appetitive system, and the medial hypothalamus and central gray matter are parts of the network for defensive behavior (Table 1-2).

Table 1-2. Goal-directed locomotion

GOALS

Exploratory: Basal ganglia

Appetitive: Lateral hypothalamic region

Defensive: Medial hypothalamus and central gray matter

Goals are interactive with cortical input: Cortical discharge is the result of the interplay between feedback and feed-forward activity. Motor cortex function ranges from subtle control modification to complete control of locomotor activity.

Further clues are again provided by studies of the cat. If the caudate nuclei are ablated bilaterally, cats exhibit a "compulsory approach syndrome." There is a tendency to approach, follow, and stick to the investigator or moving object presented to the cat. Subsequent walking is highly stimulus bound, and any obstacle or impending danger arrests the movement. The caudate is an input nucleus of the basal ganglia that also receives afferents from sensory cortex.

What then is the role of cortex? Because patients with frontal lobe lesions exhibit gait disorders, a frontal center for gait ignition and control is likely. Changes in discharges of motor cortical neurons form part of the descending signal responsible for encoding the appropriate changes in the flexor muscle activity that underlie the modifications of limb trajectory. Different populations of motor cortical cells regulate the activities of muscles that act around different joints active at different times in the swing phase of the step cycle.

The neural mechanisms underlying the control of locomotion are usually explained by separating the role of spinal circuits responsible for producing the base rhythm and descending signals responsible for modifying and fine-tuning this signal. In the intact animal, one cannot consider the activity of the spinal circuits in isolation from afferent feedback and descending signals. Cortical discharges during unobstructed locomotion form part of the signal responsible for the base rhythm. In the natural, constantly varying environment, the discharge of the motor cortical neurons is the result of interplay between the central and peripheral feedback signals ascending from the spinal cord and a feed-forward signal that provides information about the environment. Microstimulation studies of the motor cortex or pyramidal tract demonstrate that the cortex is also capable of resetting step cycle activity independent of the phase. The motor cortex control of gait may range from subtle modifications through complete control of the locomotor activity needed when walking over uneven ground or hunting prey.

SUGGESTED READING

Dickinson MH, Farley CT, Full RJ, et al. How animals move: an integrative view. Science 2000;288:100.

Dietz, V. Neurophysiology of gait disorders: present and future applications. Elect Clin Neuro 1997;103:333.

Dietz V, Duysens J. Significance of lode receptor input during locomotion: a review. Gait Posture 2000;11:102.

Drew T, Jiang W, Kably B, Lavoie S. Role of the motor cortex in the control of visually triggered gait modifications. Can J Physiol Pharmacol 1996;74:426.

Graham-Brown T. The fundamental activity of the nervous centers. J Physiol 1914;48:1846.

Grillner S, Parker D, El Manira A. Vertebrate locomotion—a Lamprey perspective. Ann NY Acad Sci 1998;860:1.

Jordan LM. Initiation of locomotion in mammals. Ann NY Acad Sci 1998;860:83.

McCrea DA. Neuronal basis of afferent-evoked enhancement of locomotor activity. Ann NY Acad Sci 1998; 860:216.

Mori S, Matsui T, Kuze B, et al. Cerebellar-induced locomotion: reticulospinal control of spinal rhythm generating mechanism in cats. Ann NY Acad Sci 1998;860:94.

Mori S, Matsuyama K, Kohyama J, et al. The constituents of postural and locomotor control systems and their interaction in cats. Brain Dev 1992;14S:S109.

Sherrington CS. The Integrative Action of the Nervous System 1906. New Haven, CT: Yale University Press.

Shik ML, Orlovsky GN. Neurophysiology of locomotor automatism. Physiol Rev 1976;56:465.

Sinnamon HM. Preoptic and hypothalamic neurons and the initiation of locomotion in the anesthetized rat. Prog Neurobiol 1993;41:323.

Whelan PJ. Control of locomotion in the decerebrate cat. Prog Neurobiol 1996;49:481.

Woollacott MH, Shumway-Cook A. Changes in posture control across the lifespan—a systems approach. Physical Therapy 1990;12:799.

Weakness

Weakness in the lower limbs is a common cause of gait disability. The distribution of weakness determines the type of gait disability and gives a clue as to the site of pathology. Broadly speaking, one can divide the causes of weakness into upper motor neuron and lower motor neuron dysfunction. The upper motor neuron extends from cortex to anterior horn cell. The lower motor neuron comprises the motor apparatus from and including the anterior horn cell to muscle.

UPPER MOTOR NEURON WEAKNESS

The Gait

Weakness in the legs in patients with upper motor neuron lesions (UMN) may be unilateral or bilateral but is most pronounced in the hip flexors, foot and toe dorsiflexors, in the hamstrings, and in the thigh abductors.

If unilateral hip flexion weakness is severe, especially with associated foot/toe dorsiflexor weakness, the foot cannot be lifted sufficiently for the toes to clear the ground and the avoiding maneuver is circumduction at the hip. The foot is therefore propelled forward in a wide lateral circle to prevent the toe from contact with the ground; this response is often not entirely successful and the toes may scrape the ground. The gait is "low stepping." The quadriceps is relatively spared, the knee can be locked, and the patient can bear weight. The soles of shoes wear out anteriorly and laterally. The toes snag on rugs or irregular spots on the ground leading to trips and falls.

If the weakness is bilateral the patient can no longer circumduct, and the toes on each side tend to scrape the floor. The gait is narrow based and scuffing, there is no start hesitation, but stride length is usually a little shortened.

Upper motor neuron weakness is usually accompanied by spasticity, which in part helps to lock the knee and allow for weight bearing.

When the weakness is subtle it may be sufficient to impair the gait and cause falls, which will be picked up only by careful examination; the patient complains of "lack of balance" but usually cannot be more specific.

The Signs

One can test muscle strength with the muscle at maximum contraction, having moved the joint to its maximum excursion, or starting midway through a movement. The examiner should become familiar with one form of testing and use that exclusively, to allow for reproducibility from examination to examination.

We are concerned here with testing strength in the lower limbs. Naturally large, strong muscles and small, weak muscles need to be evaluated. For large muscles, say the hip flexors, a good deal of power must be exerted by the examiner to test the function of the muscle. Conversely, for toe flexion or extension, the examiner will use only finger strength to oppose the movement.

Hip flexion is best tested at midposition with the patient supine; quadriceps, foot, and toe dorsiflexion, as well as toe plantar flexion, are evaluated at maximum contraction. Hamstrings are tested with the knees bent to a right angle, and thigh abductors are tested with the patient lying on the side and abducting the uppermost thigh against resistance of the examiner, which needs to be considerable to overcome the muscles.

Clearly, if muscles vary in strength from site to site, it may be difficult to assess what is "normal." *If the examiner can overcome the power of the muscle, exerting resistance close to the joint that it moves and using an equivalent muscle of his or her own* (e.g., fingers to test toe strength), *then that muscle is graded as "weak."*

The most widely used grading system to record muscle strength employs five grades, ranging from 0, or paralysis, through 5, which is normal strength. Grade 1 is a flicker of volitional movement, 2 represents the ability to move a joint to when gravity is eliminated, 3 represents the ability to move the joint against the power of gravity, and 4 simply represents weakness. Grade 4 covers a fairly wide spread of muscle power and needs to be expanded. The simplest expansion is simply to use the words *mild, moderate,* or *severe* when recording grade 4 weakness, but some physicians expand the grade by adding further numbers.

In upper motor neuron weakness, the tendon reflexes are likely increased, but the plantar responses are variable. An extensor plantar response, or Babinski response, indicates pyramidal tract dysfunction. A pure pyramidal tract lesion causes weakness, flaccidity, and a Babinski response. Hypertonia or spasticity and hyperreflexia are produced by dysfunction in nonpyramidal motor descending pathways. Spasticity and hyperreflexia in varying combination with weakness and pyramidal dysfunction represents the upper motor neuron syndrome.

Localization

Having established a pattern of upper motor neuron weakness in the legs to account for a gait disorder, the next task is to localize the site of pathology. In essence, we are attempting to find a level of dysfunction within the central motor neuraxis.

Unilateral weakness implies dysfunction in the contralateral brain, if the lesion is above the pyramidal decussation. Small lesions close to or in the motor cortex result in fairly restricted weakness in face or arm or leg. Parasagittal localization affects primarily the leg and results in a gait disorder on the basis of weakness. As the descending motor fibers approach the internal capsule and are bunched to-gether, even small lesions cause widespread weak-ness and there is loss of the exquisite somatotopic topography of the cortex. Therefore, a tiny lacunar infarct in the capsule itself can cause a dense con-tralateral hemiplegia. Lesions involving descending motor tracts in the brain stem can be localized by dysfunction of adjacent cranial nerves. Since the cranial nerves supply the ipsilateral structures and the motor tract supplies the contralateral body, a so-called crossed-hemiplegia or alternating hemiplegia results. The combination of weakness and ataxia, "ataxic hemiparesis," is a classical lacunar syndrome and usually localizes to the pons, posterior limb of internal capsule, or corona radiata.

Bilateral upper motor neuron weakness suggests a lesion in the spinal cord or myelopathy. Dysfunc-tion at a high level in the cord can produce any com-bination of upper motor neuron weakness below that level. Intramedullary or extramedullary pathol-ogy with pressure effects on the cord may result in static or progressive dysfunction in the descending and ascending long tracts, which are said to show a somatotopic orientation of fibers. Furthermore, dysfunction can be "spotty." The net result is that it is difficult to predict a level of segmental cord pathology based only on the long tract signs in the lower limbs.

The only reliable signs that allow for segmental localization are those related to root dysfunction. Thus, weakness in a myotome—that is, in a segmental lower motor neuron pattern—points to root dysfunction at that level. This is fairly easily evaluated in cervical segments (Table 2-1) but it may be impossible to demonstrate segmental weakness in the trunk. Here Beevor's sign can be helpful—on neck and trunk flexion the umbilicus may be seen to move upward to the rib cage with lower motor neuron weakness below a T10 level or deviate to the side opposite lesion at T10.

A dropped reflex in the upper limbs may be the definitive pointer to cervical radiculopathy. On the sensory side, loss of sensation in the arms in dermatomal distribution again points to cervical radiculopathy.

If a segmental level of dysfunction in the cervical or thoracic cord is suggested by the presence of root signs, imaging may be directed specifically at that level. If no level is found, the entire spinal cord must be imaged to define the pathology. It is clinically useful to differentiate spinal cord pathology into surgical pathology, which is a mechanical cause amenable to surgery, or medical pathology, which is not amenable to surgical intervention. Imaging is crucial to the differential diagnosis, and magnetic resonance imaging (MRI) is the best choice.

Table 2-1. Cervical segmental levels

Segmental Level	Muscle(s)	Action
C4	Supra-infraspinatus	First 10° of shoulder abduction Externally rotates arm
C5	Deltoid Biceps/brachioradialis	Abducts shoulder Flexes elbow
C6, C7	Triceps Brachioradialis	Extends elbow Flexes elbow in ½ supination
C6	Extensor carpi radialis	Radial wrist extension
C7	Extensor digitorum	Extends fingers
C8	Flexor digitorum	Flexes fingers
T1	Interossei Abductor dig V	Abducts fingers Abducts little finger

Note: This is a somewhat schematic representation of the main segmental innervation of the muscles of the upper limbs. It is clinically useful in localizing a single radicular level.

If we were to be absolutely anatomically correct, since virtually all muscles are of multisegmental innervation, clinical localization would be more complicated and imprecise.

If a cervical level is diagnosed, the commonest cause of cervical myelopathy in the elderly population is cervical spondylosis with cervical stenosis.

Unilateral weakness in upper motor neuron distribution in a lower limb may present more of a diagnostic challenge. Here, the crux of the problem is to decide, at the bedside, whether the pathology is above or below foramen magnum. Cervical cord pathology can cause unilateral lower limb weakness, but the finding of focal signs relating to the brain stem, upper motor neuron facial weakness, or cortical signs suggest that the brain be imaged; again MRI is the method of choice.

LOWER MOTOR NEURON WEAKNESS

The Gait

The gait will vary depending on the site of maximum weakness:

Proximal weakness. Weakness in the limb girdle leads to a *waddling* gait. With each step the contralateral pelvis tilts downward because of weakness of the ipsilateral gluteus medius. This imparts an unnatural "waddle" to the gait—normally, the contralateral pelvis tilts upward with each step, as weight is taken on the limb as gluteus contacts.

Distal weakness. The most important function of the distal leg muscles in walking is to extend the foot and toes so that with each step the toes clear the ground and do not catch or scuff. If there is weakness of foot extension and proximal muscles are strong, the hip flexors will compensate without the need for circumduction, and this results in the high stepping gait of *foot drop*, which may be bilateral or unilateral. With each step the foot flexes passively at the ankle but the toes clear the ground because of adequate hip flexion.

"In between." Quadriceps weakness produces no noticeable or characteristic gait disorder, but patients with weakness of knee extension tend to fall. Normally, with each step the knee must be locked for the limb to bear weight. If weight is taken with the knee even slightly flexed, and quadriceps is weak, the limb will buckle and the patient falls. Quadriceps weakness may cause the patient to complain of difficulty getting up or down steps or difficulty getting up from a chair.

End-plate weakness. The characteristic of neuromuscular junction weakness is fatigability. Fatigability may affect any muscle in the lower limb causing concomitant weakness during activity. The gait in myasthenia is therefore nonspecific and variable, in terms of both site and degree of weakness.

In general, in lower motor neuron weakness, the gait is narrow based, there is no start hesitation or staggering, and stride length is maintained.

The Bladder

A history of urinary bladder dysfunction is important both intrinsically and functionally and can help in differentiating upper motor neuron from more peripheral lesions. Myelopathy, in general, causes a small, spastic irritable bladder that reflects as frequency, urgency, and urgency incontinence. Thoracic myelopathy may cause bladder dyssynergia, the fundus of the bladder contracts on a closed sphincter resulting in hesitancy and retention. Cauda equina dysfunction (implying bilateral radicular dysfunction of sacral myotomes) in the acute phase causes retention.

The Signs

The lower motor neuron is part of the peripheral nervous system and weakness may have its origin in pathology at any level from anterior horn cell to muscle itself; the objective of the physical examination is to localize the source of weakness.

The technique of power testing, in general, is as described in the discussion of upper motor neuron weakness. Apart from testing thigh abduction weakness (gluteus maximus) with the patient lying on his or her side, one should test the power of the gluteus medius by observing the direction of pelvic tilt when standing on one leg (Trendelenburg's test).

The segmental innervation of the various muscles in the limbs is given in Table 2-2. The tendon reflexes in lower motor neuron problems are likely to be absent or at least depressed. The plantar responses are flexor.

Localization

In the lower limbs, it can be difficult to differentiate upper motor neuron weakness from L5 root dysfunction. Both cause weakness of foot and toe dorsiflexion, of hamstring, and of thigh abduction. The absence of hip flexion weakness and the presence of atrophy point to root dysfunction. In addition, spasticity, hyperreflexia, and an extensor plantar support a UMN diagnosis and their absence implies the reverse.

Inspection of the lower limbs may reveal atrophy or fasciculations. The distribution of atrophy gives the clue to the level of the lesion—atrophy of extensor digitorum brevis, a pure L5 muscle, on the dorsolateral aspect of the foot suggests either a lesion of the common peroneal nerve, an L5 root lesion, or far less likely, pathology in between (plexus or sciatic nerve). Atrophy of quadriceps suggests a femoral nerve lesion, a lesion in plexus,

Table 2-2. Lumbar segmental levels

Segmental Level	Muscle(s)	Action
L1, L2	Iliopsoas	Hip flexion
L3	Adductor longus Adductor brevis Adductor magnus Adductor minimus	Hip adduction
L3, L4	Quadriceps	Knee flexion
L4	Tibialis anterior	Ankle extension
L5	Extensor hallucis longus Extensor hallucis brevis Extensor digitorum longus Extensor digitorum brevis	Toe extension
	Gluteus medius	Hip abduction
L5, S1	Semitendinosis Semimembranosis Biceps femoris	Knee flexion
S1	Gastrocnemius Soleus	Ankle flexion
	Flexor digitorum brevis	Toe flexion

Note: This is a somewhat schematic representation of the main segmental innervation of the muscles of the lower limbs. It is clinically useful in localizing a single radicular level.

If we were to be absolutely anatomically correct, since virtually all muscles are of multisegmental innervation, clinical localization would be more complicated and imprecise.

or a high lumbar radiculopathy. Fasciculations are spontaneous contractions of motor units seen as irregular, short-lived, small contractions of parts of muscle under the skin. These are commonly seen in progressive anterior horn cell disease and frequently in quadriceps in patients with femoral neuropathy or diabetic amyotrophy.

In the diagnosis of the cause of *unilateral foot drop*, associated weakness helps. If there is weakness of both foot inversion and eversion, a root lesion at L5 is suspected, particularly if there is also weakness of hamstring and thigh abduction. The most common cause of lumbar radiculopathy is lumbar disc prolapse or spinal stenosis. If there is isolated weakness of foot dorsiflexion, toe extension, and foot eversion but not inversion, the likely site of pathology is in the common peroneal nerve the head of the fibula. Nerve conduction studies will confirm the site of pathology.

Bilateral foot drop, particularly if chronic, suggests the diagnosis of a degenerative disease, such as hereditary sensory/motor neuropathy, and genotyping can establish the diagnosis. If the bilateral foot drop is of acute onset, consider more the diagnosis of an acute or subacute polyneuropathy. Again, electromyography (EMG) and nerve conduction studies are very helpful.

Some simple clinical rules help with the diagnosis of *quadriceps weakness*. Isolated quadriceps weakness, usually with an absent patellar reflex, suggests a femoral nerve lesion. Weakness of thigh adduction (obturators) and hip flexion (psoas) as well as quadriceps suggests a high lumbar radiculopathy. Weakness of any two of the three muscle groups usually indicates a plexopathy. Localization can be confirmed by EMG, but whatever the localization, diabetes is a strong contender in the differential diagnosis of weakness in quadriceps. Imaging of pelvis and lumbar spine usually is indicated.

Pelvic girdle weakness with a waddling gait suggests particular diligence in testing strength in the shoulder girdle and neck flexors and extensors. Weakness in these muscles supports the notion of "proximal" weakness, which in turn suggests a clinical diagnosis of myopathy and rarely a myasthenic syndrome (Lambert-Eaton syndrome). The investigations of choice are a blood creatine phosphokinase (CPK) and EMG. Support from the laboratory tests then indicate muscle biopsy to make a definitive diagnosis.

Intermittent weakness in the lower limbs suggests a diagnosis of myasthenia. The association of intermittent weakness in the lower limbs together with intermittent dysfunction of the upper limbs and diplopia or bulbar dysfunction might support the notion. The clinical test for end-plate disease is the demonstration of weakness precipitated by exercise, a myasthenic reaction. End-plate studies in the EMG department usually clinch the diagnosis.

Motor neuron disease (MND) can present as a progressive gait disorder. Weakness may initially seem to be myotomal and unilateral but becomes diffuse within 6–12 months and is associated with widespread atrophy, fasciculations, hyperreflexia, and sometimes extensor plantar responses. If initial workup is negative, the best test is that of "time"— all will be revealed. Laboratory investigations for motor neuron disease include a blood CPK, an EMG and MRI imaging to be quite sure there is no other pathology, which might be more treatable— thus cervical spondylosis can mimic the syndrome and is very treatable. If the presentation is entirely lower motor neuron, without hyperreflexia and extensor plantar responses, the diagnosis may be progressive muscular atrophy (PMA), a variant of MND. The syndrome of motor neuropathy with segmental conduction block, although rare, is a treatable cause of progressive disability and mimics PMA. The diagnosis is made by sophisticated nerve conduction studies and the finding of antibodies to peripheral myelin components in the blood. Treatment with IVIg can be very rewarding.

SUGGESTED READING

Messina C. Pathophysiology of muscle tone. Funct Neu-
    rol 1990;5:217.
Ronthal M. Weakness. In Samuels M (ed), Office Prac-
    tice of Neurology. New York: Churchill Livingstone,
    1996.
Walshe FMR. The Babinski plantar response, its form
    and its physiological and pathological significance.
    Brain 1956;79:529.
Younger DS. Differential diagnosis of progressive flaccid
    weakness. Semin Neurol 1993;13:241.

Deafferentation

Proper functioning of a motor system requires not only motor *output* but also sensory *input* to allow monitoring of the desired effect. Loss of this feedback system can be devastating for the mechanics of gait. The critical feedback system is that of proprioception or position sense. Loss of pinprick, temperature, light touch, or of vibration sense, while uncomfortable, is not likely to cause a marked deterioration in gait. Spinocerebellar feedback is of theoretical importance but it is hard to demonstrate that dysfunction in these feedback systems, except in the hereditary spinocerebellar ataxias, is a frequent or potent cause of gait dysfunction.

Proprioceptive loss can be secondary to pathology in either the peripheral or central nervous system, and the approach to clinical localization is therefore akin to that used to determine the level in the neuraxis of a source of weakness. The divide between central and peripheral pathology is sometimes not all that obvious at the bedside, and the disordered gait of proprioceptive loss is similar whatever the level of lesion.

Mechanoreceptors for proprioception are present in the skin, the joints, and the muscle spindles. They represent some of the most distal part of the nervous system. Information is carried centrally in large, myelinated, fast-conducting fibers of mixed nerves. The afferent fibers, whose cell bodies lie in the dorsal root ganglia enter the spinal cord via the dorsal root and synapse in the dorsal column nuclei. Proprioceptive fibers then travel cranially in the dorsal columns of the spinal cord and enter the medial leminiscus in the brain stem, synapsing for the second time in the ventral posterior lateral nucleus and posterior nuclei of the thalamus. These cells in turn project in the corona radiata to the posterior parietal cortex. Dysfunction at any level in the system can cause proprioceptive loss and gait dysfunction.

THE GAIT

The classical description of a tabetic gait (bilateral severe proprioception deficit) is "high-stepping and stamping." The notion is that stamping the feet increases sensory feedback and overcomes the deficit in proprioceptive function. The gait is slightly wide based, stride length is normal or a little reduced, and the gait deteriorates markedly in the dark, when it may become frankly ataxic and reeling. More commonly we see patients deliberately striking the ground with the heel and then placing the foot with somewhat of a soft and deliberate "slap."

THE SIGNS

Position sense is usually tested in the great toes—the toe is immobilized but for the distal joint and the distal phalanx is grasped with a side-to-side pressure by the examiner's fingers to eliminate pressure cues. The distal phalanx is then moved up or down starting with 1° excursions, and the subject, with eyes closed, is asked to report on the final position—up or down. Appreciation of movement may be tested by making subtle adjustments in toe posture and asking for the direction of movement or presence of movement itself. In the most severe cases, position sense will be defective even for ankle joint movements.

For testing proprioception in the upper limbs, a similar technique is employed. The patient is asked to report on small excursions of the most distal phalanx of a finger. In the finger-to-finger test, one arm is passively moved and brought to rest in a random position with the forefinger extended. The subject is then asked to touch that extended forefinger with the forefinger of the other hand. Failure of the fingers to meet with the eyes closed but normal coordination with the eyes open indicates proprioceptive dysfunction.

The patient is then asked to stand with the feet closed on narrow base. When the subject's eyes are closed, one observes for swaying, usually in the lateral direction, a positive Romberg's sign. The test is positive only if the patient is stable with the eyes open and sways with the eyes closed.

The usual tests for cerebellar ataxia, the finger nose, or and heel shin test discussed in the chapter on ataxia may be mildly abnormal. If these tests are carried out with the eyes open and then closed and there is marked deterioration when the patient is not actively visually monitoring the movement, the ataxia is likely to be due to proprioceptive dysfunction, so-called sensory ataxia.

One can test skin proprioceptors by stimulating the skin with a blunt object that is scraped upward or downward on the leg (trunk or arm), and the patient is asked to identify the direction of movement with the eyes closed.

Patients with loss of position sense in the hands may exhibit pseudoathetosis. With the eyes closed, ask the patient to hold the arms extended horizontally in front. The patient with severe proprioceptive loss may demonstrate aimless spontaneous movements of the fingers or even wrists when visual feedback is eliminated.

LOCALIZATION

When the large fibers in the peripheral nerves are involved as part of a peripheral neuropathy, small fibers are usually also involved in the process. Therefore, in patients who have proprioceptive loss as part of a diffuse polyneuropathy, there is almost always stocking/glove sensory loss for pinprick and temperature as well. The tendon reflexes generally are absent, indicating a peripheral process. Involvement of motor fibers is variable, and they may be spared. The commonest cause of peripheral neuropathy with profound sensory loss is diabetes, so-called diabetic pseudotabes, but in general, a widespread search for underlying systemic disease causing peripheral neuropathy must be initiated.

When the pathology is primarily within the dorsal root ganglia, there is no clear distal-to-proximal gradient of sensory loss. Widespread are-flexia accompanies a usually profound loss of position sense and vibration sense. Onset is occasionally acute and autoimmune but more often is insidious and chronic, which indicates a search for occult neoplasm as the initiator. Other rare causes are pyridoxin toxicity and the anti-myelin-associated-glycoprotein antibody syndrome.

The prototype clinical syndrome of posterior column dysfunction in the spinal cord is tabes dorsalis due to tertiary syphilis. These patients have a high stepping gait, absent ankle jerks, and sometimes extensor plantar responses if the infection is widespread in the brain and causes *taboparesis*. They may complain of sudden shooting pains in root distribution, the "lightning pains" of tabes. Because of joint deafferentation, severe progressive painless osteoarthritis with joint disorganization can occur—Charcot joints. The clue to the diagnosis may be the finding of light/near dissociation in the pupillary light reflexes. Nowadays, syphilis is rare and other pathology is more likely. Myelopathy on a mechanical basis may be due to intrinsic cord pathology or extrinsic cord compression.

The presence of Lhermitte's sign—tingly paresthesiae radiating down the arms, spine, and legs, precipitated by neck flexion—localizes the posterior column dysfunction to the cervical cord and suggests the diagnosis of multiple sclerosis. Other cord pathology is not excluded, and the symptom could as likely be produced by a cervical disc or cervical stenosis with cord compression. Subacute combined degeneration due to vitamin B12 deficiency is an unlikely candidate for pure posterior column dysfunction but should be considered if the patient presents with paresthesiae in the hands, absent ankle jerks, and extensor plantar responses.

If the diagnosis is unclear, imaging the spinal cord is mandatory; and if the imaging does not give the answer, the spinal fluid should be examined.

On occasion, patients are seen with loss of position sense in the fingers, intact or mildly affected proprioception in the toes, yet with a gait disorder on the basis of motor tract dysfunction. Loss of position sense in the fingers only strongly suggests a very high cervical or foramen magnum area lesion. This is sometimes called *reversed* dissociated sensory loss. Likely pathologies at the craniovertebral junction include a foramen magnum meningioma, Chiari malformation, or basilar invagination. Loss of position sense and vibration sense limited to the upper limbs and upper torso is suggestive of lesion at the decussation of the medial leminiscus. These patients may also show upper motor neuron signs in the upper limbs only and loss of vibration sense over the clavicles.

The medial medullary syndrome is extremely rare, but an infarct in this area can result in loss of posterior column sensation together with upper motor neuron signs on the opposite side of the body. The clue to the level is ipsilateral tongue paralysis.

Thalamic lesions rarely cause isolated proprioceptive loss, rather loss of all modalities of sensation on the contralateral side of the body is the rule.

Lastly, cortical lesions in the parietal lobe may have loss of position sense as part of the clinical complex.

SUGGESTED READING

Collins WF, Nulsen FE, Randt CT. Relationship of peripheral nerve fiber size and sensation in man. Arch Neurol 1960;3:381.

Cook AW, Browder EJ. Function of posterior columns in man. Arch Neurol 1965;12:72.

McCloskey DI. Kinesthetic sensibility. Physiol Rev 1978; 58:763.

Vestibular Dysfunction, Dizziness

A common complaint of patients with gait disorders is dizziness, or loss of balance. The main sources of information about the position of the head and body in space are the vestibular system and visual and proprioceptive input. Dysfunction in any of these input systems can result in a feeling of dizziness, which represents a mismatch in the afferent information received by the brain. The patient can rarely distinguish which afferent system is out of kilter, but diagnosis can usually be made at the bedside following an exquisitely detailed history and examination.

The word *dizziness* can be regarded as a repository for multiple symptoms with various interpretations. Some physicians try to differentiate dizziness

45

from "true vertigo," implying that the latter appella-
tion means a sensation of spinning. For purposes of
this discussion, vertigo and dizziness are regarded as
somewhat synonymous, both implying a feeling or
illusion of movement or disorientation in space, a
sensation of linear displacement or tilt, or simply
loss of balance or dysequilibrium.

It is important to distinguish between vestibular
and nonvestibular causes of dizziness (Table 4-1).

Table 4-1. Dizziness

Dizziness is a nonspecific complaint

Vestibular dizziness
    Almost always episodic
    Subjective sensation of spinning
    Compensation usually occurs in weeks, but bilateral
        vestibulopathy is a cause of chronic gait disorder
    Nystagmus is prominent
        Vestibulopathy

Nonvestibular dizziness
    Lightheaded, floaty sensation, just "loss of balance"
        Hypotension
        Arrhythmia
        Neck spasm
        Seizure
        Ocular
        Psychogenic

CAUSES OF DIZZINESS

Vestibular Dizziness

A feeling of spinning usually indicates vestibular dysfunction, is almost always episodic, and is often accompanied by nausea and vomiting. Associated hearing loss, or tinnitus, strengthens the case for a vestibular cause. During attacks of acute unilateral peripheral vestibular dysfunction, the patient may have an ataxic gait, but the symptoms rarely last more than 2 weeks and, even if the pathology persists, compensation occurs fairly rapidly. Gradually progressive vestibular dysfunction usually causes a nondescript feeling of dizziness rather than rotary vertigo. Bilateral chronic vestibular dysfunction may cause a severe gait ataxia.

Nonvestibular Dizziness

Nonvestibular dizziness, may be described as a feeling of lightheadedness, a floating sensation, or just plain loss of balance; and it has a multitude of causes. Precipitating factors, information gleaned from the history, can help with the differential diagnosis. For example, a feeling of lightheadedness and loss of balance present only in the upright position could represent the symptoms of postural hypotension.

Physiological Dizziness

Almost everyone, at one time or another, has experienced physiological vestibular vertigo, and so the sensation produced by mild vestibular dysfunction should be easy to recognize. As children, we play games that involve spinning around or play on roundabouts. As adults, we may experience seasickness. In all these situations, there is a feeling of subjective movement or tilting and, often, spinning, with veering to one side on walking. There may be varying degrees of nausea and vomiting. In seasickness, there is a classical mismatch between what the vestibular apparatus signals and what the subject sees, and to minimize that mismatch, we are told to go on deck and watch the horizon.

VESTIBULAR FUNCTION

The semicircular canals are sensitive to *angular* acceleration of the head in space. Angular movements of the head cause a displacement of endolymph, which in turn displaces the cupulae. The initial deviation of the cupula is related to the constant acceleration stimulus, but when the stimulus is terminated, the cupula returns to the resting position—a pendulum-like movement. This movement generates an electrical nerve potential proportionate to the stimulus.

The maculae in the saccule and utricle contain the otolith organs, which are sensitive to *linear* head acceleration and gravity. The nerve fibers innervating the maculae are activated by changes in position of the head in space.

Vestibular reflexes allow for normal gait and posture. The body must resist the pull of gravity or it would collapse to the ground. Vestibular reflex activity arising from the maculae induces muscle contraction to compensate for steady changes in the direction of the force of gravity. At the same time, during movement, the head and eyes must be kept stable and transitory compensatory contractions of muscles to maintain equilibrium and ocular stability during head movement are generated by both the semicircular canals during angular acceleration and the otoliths during linear acceleration. Both organs are active in the reflex maintenance of generalized muscular tone. The vestibular-ocular reflex is an open-loop system controlling a viscous load, the eyeball. The vestibular-colic reflex is a closed-loop reflex with a predominantly inertial load, the head. Neck muscles are more sluggish than extraocular muscles.

The primary vestibular nerve enters the brain stem and, via ascending and descending branches, connects with the vestibular nuclei and the cerebellum to relay complex information about the position and movement of the head in space. The vestibular nuclei also receive information from the cervical muscles, the cerebellum, the reticular formation, the spinal cord, and the contralateral vestibular nuclei. The output is to the extraocular muscles, the spinal cord, and somatic muscles, also to thalamus and cortex.

Normal tone in somatic antigravity muscles is the result of a fine balance between stimulation and inhibition. The major facilitatory sources are the lateral vestibular nuclei and the rostral reticular formation. The major inhibitory centers are cortex, basal ganglia, cerebellum, and caudal reticular formation. The vestibulothalamocortical projections integrate vestibular, proprioceptive, and visual signals to provide a conscious awareness of body orientation.

Input from the peripherally distributed balance organs is balanced. Imbalance results in a slow deviation of eyes directed toward the site of lesion. Rapid correction of this slow drift results in the fast phase of nystagmus. Similarly, imbalance of peripheral (and central) input may result in incoordination of upper limb, trunk, and lower limb muscles. Thus, disturbances in input and integration of signals recording movement and position of the head in space can result in disturbances of posture and gait or an illusion of movement. If there is nystagmus, the patient may complain that visually observed objects are moving or jiggling, *oscillopsia*. Unilateral dysfunction may result in a complaint that visual objects seem to be moving in the direction opposite to that of the slow phase of nystagmus, and an illusion of linear movement or tilting suggests isolated involvement of the otolith or its central connections.

THE GAIT

The severity of signs and symptoms varies. The patient may complain only of a feeling of imbalance or symptoms may escalate to a complaint of severe spinning or rotation.

In concert, the gait disturbance varies from an occasional stumble through veering to one or other side and then frank ataxia. In general, the legs are slightly spread to give a wide base. With unilateral dysfunction the patient will veer toward the pathological side and may stumble to that side. Stride length is slightly shortened. With bilateral disease, the gait is frankly ataxic but almost never to the extent seen in patients with cerebellar dysfunction.

THE SIGNS

Ears

Evaluation of the vestibular system in the patient with dizziness begins with an examination of the ear itself. The eardrum is inspected for scarring, opacity, perforation, or other local pathology, such as a glomus or hemorrhage. Hearing is tested using a finger rub on each side. One can whisper numbers or language to test for speech discrimination (lost early in vestibular schwannomas) and the tuning fork can be used to discriminate between air conduction and bone conduction hearing loss (Rinne test and Weber's test).

Eyes

On prolonged lateral gaze, jerky movements of the eyeballs indicate nystagmus. Nystagmus with a slow and quick phase is suggestive of vestibular or vestibular connection dysfunction. Nystagmus may be spontaneous, gaze evoked, or positional. The vestibular system, which receives input from both ears, is the main source of oculomotor tonus, and unbalanced input results in drift interrupted by fast components in the opposite direction. Although the majority of patients with vestibular dysfunction have peripheral pathology, central pathology in the brain stem or an acute cerebellar lesion can also cause vestibular dysfunction. The character of the nystagmus can help with localization.

In *spontaneous nystagmus*, vertical and torsional components, a change in direction (nystagmus on both left and right gaze with a change in direction of the slow and quick phase), lack of inhibition by fixation, and focal signs relating to the brain stem indicate a central source. Unilateral spontaneous nystagmus is almost always peripheral in origin.

In *gaze-evoked nystagmus*, the eyes are unable to maintain stable conjugate deviation away from the primary position and drift back toward the center, and corrective fast saccades reset the desired gaze position. Bidirectional gaze-evoked nystagmus suggests a central source, and persistent nystagmus to one side only usually indicates a peripheral source.

Positional nystagmus is that seen when the head is placed in a specific relation to gravity. This is usually peripheral in origin, and Hallpike's maneuver is used to elicit the sign. The patient is instructed to keep the eyes open, rather than closed (which is the natural inclination to minimize visual/vestibular mismatch and diminish the sensation of spinning). With the patient supine, the head is tilted 30° below the horizontal and twisted to one side or the other. In benign paroxysmal positional vertigo (BPPV), there is a short latent period, then a limited episode of a rotary nystagmus, which spontaneously fatigues. If there is no latent period and no fatigue, the positional nystagmus may be of either peripheral or central origin, but the signs do not support a diagnosis of BPPV.

Upper Limbs

Past pointing is the term used to describe a reactive deviation of the extremities caused by an imbalance in the vestibular system. The patient is asked to place his or her index finger on the tip of the examiner's index finger, to close the eyes, raise the arm to a vertical position, then return to the initial starting point. Recurrent deviation to one side is past pointing. While the test can be strikingly positive, the result should not be considered in isolation, and extra labyrinthine contributions should be eliminated as far as possible. The regular finger nose test, as discussed in the chapter on ataxia, does not identify past pointing, because proprioceptive feedback allows for accurate localization even in the absence of normal vestibular function.

Trunk

The patient is asked to stand with the feet together as in performing Romberg's test for proprioceptive loss. Vestibular dysfunction may result in instability of the trunk and lower limbs with swaying or falling to one side. Patients with acute unilateral labyrinthine lesions sway and fall toward the diseased side, in the direction of the slow component of nystagmus. The test is not invariably positive, and sometimes patients sway toward the "wrong" side. A "sharpened" Romberg's test may be more sensitive. The patient stands with feet aligned in a tandem heel-toe position with the eyes closed and the arms folded. Normal subjects under the age of 70 should be able to maintain this position for 30 seconds or more.

Lower Limbs

With the eyes closed, the patient is asked to walk forward or to take about 50 steps on the spot. Patients with the vestibular dysfunction tend to turn in the direction of past pointing and fall, again in the direction of the slow phase of nystagmus (Unterberger and Fukuda tests).

Tandem gait walking with the eyes open is essentially a test of cerebellar function, vision compensates for vestibular and proprioceptive deficits, but acute severe vestibular deficits may interfere with tandem gait walking. Provided cerebellar function and proprioceptive function is intact, tandem gait walking with closed eyes is a good test of the vestibular function. With eyes closed and the arms folded across the chest the subject is asked to take 10 steps forward. The number of steps taken without side stepping is scored in three successive trials, and most normals can make a minimum of 10 accurate tandem steps in three trials. The direction of falling is not a reliable lateralizer of the vestibular dysfunction.

Causes of Vertigo

Peripheral vertigo is usually episodic, and in the differential diagnosis of vestibulopathy, one should consider acute vestibular neuronitis, Meniere's disease, and benign positional vertigo. Other causes (Table 4-2) are rare. Vestibular neuronitis, sometimes called *labyrinthitis*, is a self-limiting syndrome of severe rotary vertigo; with associated pallor, sweating, and vomiting; aggravated by head movements; and associated with unilateral nystagmus. Meniere's disease is characterized by severe recurrent episodes of peripheral vertigo with similar symptoms but also a feeling of fullness in the ear, hearing loss, and tinnitus. Vertebrobasilar insufficiency is an often-quoted cause of vertigo but is in fact extremely rare. Only if the vertigo is associated with transient brain stem signs or symptoms is this

Table 4-2. Vestibulopathy

Acute vestibular neuronitis
Meniere's disease
Benign paroxysmal positional vertigo
Drug induced
Postconcussion syndrome
Bacterial labyrinthitis
Perilymph fistula
Labyrinthine ischemia

a likely diagnosis. Likewise, vestibular schwannoma is often listed as a cause of peripheral vertigo—almost never does this tumor present with vertigo, rather it presents with hearing loss, perhaps some mild disequilibrium, which may become severe in the case of large tumors that compress the brain stem. Finally, drug-induced vertigo should never be forgotten. Alcohol, tranquilizer drugs, anticonvulsants, aminoglycoside antibiotics, and antihypertensives that could cause postural hypotension should be considered. If there is doubt or a central mechanism is seriously considered, the brain should be imaged with MRI.

NONVESTIBULAR DIZZINESS

The complaint "I am dizzy" can hide a multitude of sins. In this section, we discuss causes of imbalance and dizziness not particularly related to the vestibular system. To a greater or lesser extent, they may be associated with a subjective or, less frequently, objective gait disorder, which can vary from an occasional stumble to a usually narrow-based gait ataxia.

More often than not, even after an exquisitely detailed history, the diagnosis rests on the examination and provocative tests.

Postural Hypotension

Particularly when the complaint is related to being in an upright posture, the blood pressure should be taken in the supine and erect postures to screen for postural hypotension leading to decreased cerebral perfusion and presyncope. Associated symptoms may include sweating, pallor, and occasionally the patient has sensation of an impending faint. The blood pressure is taken supine, immediately after standing, and then a delayed standing reading is taken after 3–5 minutes. The pulse rate is measured simultaneously. Since mainly the systolic pressure relates to cerebral perfusion, use of the radial pulse as a marker is as sensitive as the usual stethoscope method. A drop in systolic blood pressure of more than 10 points on assuming an erect posture is likely to be pathological. If there is a concomitant tachycardia, it is likely that the autonomic nervous system is intact and the possibility of hypovolemia should be considered. If there is a significant fall of blood pressure in an erect posture with no compensatory tachycardia, autonomic dysfunction is diagnosed, but drug-induced beta blockade may be the cause of the lack of compensatory tachycardia. Patients with primarily peripheral autonomic failure have an immediate drop in systolic pressure on assuming an erect posture. Patients with dysfunction of central autonomic pathways may show a delayed fall after a few minutes until the peripheral stored catecholamines are depleted. Tilt table testing in the autonomic laboratory should be the next investigation of choice.

Cardiac Arrhythmia

Episodically reduced cerebral perfusion can result in episodic dizziness, presyncope or syncope, and episodic falls. A history of episodic stumbling even in the absence of a good story of palpitations and with a normal physical examination should trigger cardiac monitoring for arrhythmia.

Cervical Vertigo

A vague feeling of unsteadiness, lightheadedness, imbalance, with or without pain and stiffness in the posterior cervical muscles can be caused by cervical muscle spasm. The major afferent input to the vestibular nuclei from the neck is from proprioceptors in the paravertebral joints and capsules. Also a relatively minor but significant input comes from the paravertebral muscles. If the examination is negative for focal signs and the history is little vague, it is always worth looking at the neck. Restricted rotation, palpable posterior cervical muscle spasm, and muscle tenderness to even light palpation may be the clue to cervical vertigo. If the patient is currently symptomatic, massage of the posterior cervical muscles with the patient lying supine may temporarily alleviate the symptoms and prove the diagnosis.

Focal Seizure Disorder

Seizures arising in one or the other temporal lobe occasionally present with intermittent dizziness or even frank vertigo. The history of patients with dizziness should include an inquiry for other symptoms of simple or complex partial seizures of temporal lobe origin. A history of intermittent hallucinations of taste, smell, depersonalization, derealization, or vague abdominal symptoms might be the clue. An electroencephalogram (EEG) may help to make the diagnosis, and with a positive history, even with a negative EEG, a trial of anticonvulsant is worth considering for patients with intermittent dizziness of unknown cause.

Ocular Dizziness

Normal balance and gait is dependent on proprioceptive, vestibulocerebellar, and visual input to the motor system. Nystagmus results in oscillopsia, which may be what the patient means when the complaint is "dizziness." Furthermore, at times of refractive change, patients will frequently be a little unbalanced until compensation occurs.

Psychogenic Dizziness

The history in the dizzy patient should include questions about anxiety. The major dilemma, however, is which comes first, anxiety or dizziness.

Anxiety may provoke mild dizziness by producing spasm in cervical muscles, and patients complain of being a little off balance, perhaps with an occasional stagger.

More severe episodic dizziness, which can take the form of frank rotary vertigo, can be the presenting symptom of hyperventilation or panic attacks. The patient will usually deny frank hyperventilation but one can reproduce symptoms in the office by forced voluntary hyperventilation for about 3 minutes. After a positive provocative test, some explanation is warranted; and one should explain that mild hyperventilation over a prolonged period is the equivalent of severe overbreathing for a short time as in the provocative test.

Agoraphobia and space phobia may be associated with a complaint of dizziness.

Phobic postural vertigo is characterized by a frightening feeling of dizziness with subjective postural and gait instability. Patients describe their dizziness as a perception of illusory body motion in brief bouts lasting seconds to hours and even days, associated with anxiety and escape reactions.

Physiologic Dizziness

Motion sickness on boats and sometimes car trips is probably related to a mismatch between visual and vestibular input. Because the environment is moving with the subject and looks unchanged, visual/vestibular conflict results in a feeling of disorientation, imbalance, and frequently pallor, sweating, nausea, and vomiting. About 50% of astronauts develop motion sickness in space, probably due to a mismatch between otolith input and semicircular canals signals as well as visual signals in a gravity-free environment.

Multifactorial Dizziness

Finally, especially in older patients, dizziness may be of multifactorial origin. A combination of deafferentation, vestibular dysfunction, decreased visual acuity, and impaired hearing as well as the use of dizziness provoking drugs can summate to produce major disability. Such patients may be unable to walk without assistance.

TREATMENT

Treatment of the patient with vertigo or dizziness is largely that of the cause. Positional vertigo may respond to vestibular physical therapy and the Epley maneuver. Meniere's disease occasionally responds to a diuretic. Postural hypotension may respond to the use of support hose or drugs to keep the blood pressure stable, and cardiac arrhythmia requires specific intervention by a cardiologist. A seizure disorder almost always responds to anticonvulsant, and minor tranquilizers and psychiatric support are used for the anxious patient. If the diagnosis of cervical vertigo is made, muscle relaxants, local heat, some support at night, and gentle massage may carry the day.

There is no good "dizzy pill." Meclizine and Dramamine are anticholinergic, and since input from the vestibular apparatus is cholinergic, they are of theoretical benefit, but the automatic prescription of these motion sickness drugs usually is ineffective and the drugs are sedating. They are of some symptomatic benefit if given prior to exposure to motion. Gentle sedation with diazepam is usually more effective.

SUGGESTED READING

Baloh RW, Honrubia V, Jacobson K. Benign positional vertigo: clinical and oculographic features in 240 cases. Neurology 1987;37:371.

Bender MB. Oscillopsia. Arch Neurol 1965;13:204.

Buttner-Ennever JA. Vestibular oculomotor organization. In Fuchs AF, Becker W (eds), The Neural Control of Eye Movements. Amsterdam: Elsevier, 1981.

Dix M, Hallpike C. The pathology, symptomatology, and
diagnosis of certain common disorders of the vestibular systems. Ann Otol Rhinol Laryngol 1952;
61:987.

Drachman DA, Hart CW. An approach to the dizzy
patient. Neurology 1972;22:323.

Fregley AR. Vestibular ataxia and its measurement in man.
In Kornhuber HH (ed), Handbook of Sensory Physiology VI, Part 2. New York: Springer-Verlag, 1974.

Fukuda T. The stepping test: two phases of the labyrinthine reflex. Acta Otolaryngol 1959;50:95.

Leigh RJ, Zee DS. The Neurology of Eye Movements.
New York, Oxford: Oxford University Press, 1999.

Magerian GJ. Hyperventilation syndromes: infrequently
recognized common expressions of anxiety and
stress. Medicine 1982;61:219.

Cerebellar Ataxia

The term *ataxia* denotes lack of coordination and, in the context of gait disorders, implies lack of coordination in the legs such that normal ambulation is impaired. Probably, in everyday life, the commonest cause of gait ataxia is alcoholic intoxication.

Ataxia implies dysfunction in the cerebellum or cerebellar connections, but occasionally bifrontal disease can present with an ataxic gait of sorts. Cerebellar gait ataxia occurs only with movement. In ataxia due to deafferentation, all movements are carried out in an incoordinate fashion, modified by the aid of vision. Cerebellar ataxia is restricted to active complex movements and is not improved with vision.

The cerebellum can be regarded as an information processing center for the learning and programming of movement, regulating movement, and controlling balance by feedback mechanisms. Information about limb position and movement is supplied by the ascending spinocerebellar tracts and about the position of the head in space by vestibular afferents. After processing in cerebellar cortex, the information is relayed to the deep cerebellar nuclei and thence via the superior cerebellar peduncle to ventrolateral nucleus of thalamus and motor cortex. The cortex feeds back to cerebellum via posterior limb of internal capsule, the pons and thence back to cerebellum via the middle cerebellar peduncle. This cortico-ponto-cerebellar-thalamo-cortical circuit is a closed loop that provides feedback monitoring of pyramidal tract activity in relation to the position of the limbs; completion of the circuit in man takes about 20 milliseconds. Dysfunction anywhere along the course of the connections can result in ataxia—even frontal dysfunction can result in an ataxia of gait and can be misdiagnosed as a primary posterior fossa lesion.

The cerebellum projects back to the spinal cord via the lateral vestibular nucleus and reticular formation, which allows for control of alpha and gamma motor neurons in the cord.

THE GAIT

Adjectives used described the gait ataxia of cerebellar dysfunction include *staggering*, *reeling*, and *drunken*.

The legs are spread so that the base is wide, and the patient staggers from side to side in a zigzag fashion, being unable to walk a straight line. Stride length is slightly shortened. If the deficit is mild and subtle, the base may not be very wide, but the patient will occasionally lurch to one side or the other, miss a step, and stagger particularly on turning.

THE SIGNS

The major subdivisions of the cerebellum include the vermis and anterior lobe (paleocerebellum), the cerebellar hemispheres (neocerebellum), and the flocculonodular lobe (archicerebellum). Dysfunction in vermis results in truncal and gait ataxia, and cerebellar hemisphere dysfunction results in appendicular ataxia. Because of major connections with the vestibular system, flocculonodular dysfunction is associated with vertigo and ataxia.

TESTS FOR CEREBELLAR DYSFUNCTION

Trunk

Patients with trunk ataxia sway when sitting—the trunk muscles are incapable of coordinating their contractions in the interest of immobilization and stabilization. When standing, a light tap on the chest, back, or shoulder disturbs the patient's equilibrium and causes a stagger or fall. A patient who is disturbed while sitting on the side of the bed will sway and perhaps fall into the bed. If asked to stand with the feet together, the patient may sway to either side, forward, or backward. This disturbance of station, however, is not specific for vermis dysfunction and is seen with severe cerebellar hemisphere dysfunction as well.

Upper Limbs

The patient holds both arms extended horizontally in front and closes the eyes. In most cases of unilateral cerebellar dysfunction, the ipsilateral arm swings outward.

In the upper limbs, the "finger-nose" test demonstrates an action or intention tremor. The patient is asked to repetitively touch the examiner's finger held in front of him or her, more or less at eye or nose level, with his or her own index finger and then touch his or her nose. Because the tremor of cerebellar gait ataxia is generated in proximal muscles, the abnormality is more flagrant if the patient is asked to abduct the shoulder while performing the task. The movement begins normally but becomes tremulous, and the tremor increases in amplitude as the target is approached. The target may not be reached (hypometria) or may be missed, and the finger overshoots the examiner's finger (hypermetria). There is a disturbance of rate, regularity, and force among the individual parts of this compound movement, which results in dysmetria. On attempting to grasp an object, say a glass of water, the hand is held open in exaggerated superfluous manner before the grasp, and on release the fingers are overextended, much like the early movements of the developing child.

The patient is asked to rapidly supinate and pronate the forearms or to slap the palms and then the dorsum of the hands on the knees. The affected limb moves in an irregular fashion, and the arm deviates from its normal position (dysdiadochokinesis). Instead of asking the patient to perform alternative movements as rapidly as possible, one may ask him or her to tap a rhythmic pattern of varying complexity—incoordination in this test (arrhythmokinesis) is specific for cerebellar dysfunction and is not seen in Parkinson's disease or spasticity.

There is a delay in starting and stopping contraction: The examiner's fingers point at the patient, the palm is down and parallel to the floor. The examiner's hand is abruptly jerked upward or downward a short distance. The patient is asked to mirror the movement with his or her own hand. In the presence of cerebellar dysfunction, there is marked overshoot. The patient is asked to pull against the power of the examiner, who applies resistance to the forearm and then suddenly releases the hold. If there is cerebellar dysfunction, the patient is unable to change the pattern of contraction quickly and may even strike himself or herself before being able to halt the flexion contraction. A variant of this test is to ask the patient to hold the limb rigid while the examiner applies resistance rhythmically and alternatively in an attempt to move it. The ability to quickly adjust muscular contraction to oppose this alternatively applied resistance is lost, and the limb is easily forced out of its position.

A sample of the patient's handwriting reflects the abnormality of coordination. The script is large, particularly at the end of the word or sentence, and scraggly.

Lower Limbs

Coordination in the lower limbs is best tested by the "heel-shin test." Lying supine, the patient is asked to run the heel down the contralateral shin, placing the heel first on the knee and ending the movement at the ankle. The ataxic patient excessively flexes the leg so that the heel is placed on the thigh rather than on the knee. As the heel runs down the shin, it deviates from side to side. The patient is then asked to rhythmically tap with the heel on the shin midway between knee and ankle. The movement is performed in an irregular fashion, the heel may miss the shin at times, or if the disturbance is less severe, the metronome-like rhythm is lost.

The patient is asked to walk along a straight line. In unilateral cerebellar dysfunction, there is a tendency to homolateral deviation. In bilateral dysfunction, the gait is as described previously.

Other Manifestations

Cerebellar dysfunction is often associated with hypotonia. The patient is asked to rest the elbows on a table and hold the forearms vertically with the wrist muscles relaxed. Normally, the hand makes an angle of around 30° above the horizontal plane. When hypotonia is present, the hand approaches the horizontal or sags below it. If the thigh of the relaxed patient lying supine is rotated vigorously, the foot flails limply from side to side. If the knee jerks are tested with the legs dangling over the edge of the examination couch, the reflexes are undamped and the legs move back and forth in a pendular fashion.

Speech may be slurred and multisyllabic words are broken up to yield a scanning quality.

Nystagmus is frequent in lesions of the flocculonodular lobe but is also frequently seen in diffuse disease and brain stem dysfunction. The patient is asked to fixate on targets in the left and then a right visual field. Overshoot is called *ocular dysmetria.*

LOCALIZATION

Archicerebellar syndrome. Gait ataxia, vertigo, and nystagmus.

Paleocerebellar syndrome. Gait ataxia, lower limb incoordination, and trunk ataxia.

Neocerebellar syndrome. Hypotonia, dyssynergia, dysmetria, tremor, gait ataxia, and nystagmus.

In practice, it is frequently difficult to differentiate these syndromes one from another, and the superimposition of cranial nerve dysfunction or motor or sensory long tract signs implies brain stem localization. In the setting of a chronic cerebellar-type gait disorder, the addition of extrapyramidal signs of a parkinsonian type or pyramidal signs suggests the presence of a multisystem degenerative process.

The clinical examination defines the cause of the gait problem as being cerebellar or cerebellar connections in origin. This is the "where" of the diagnosis, it remains for the clinician to determine the pathogenesis, the "what."

CAUSES OF CEREBELLAR GAIT ATAXIA

The causes of cerebellar dysfunction are legion. Only a smattering of the differential will be discussed. Cerebellar dysfunction may be congenital or developmental, and the possibilities include platybasia, Chiari malformation, Dandy Walker malformation, and various forms of agenesis and hypoplasia of the cerebellum. Platybasia may also be acquired in later life if the bones at the base of skull soften as in Paget's disease.

Purkinje cells are particularly vulnerable to hypoxia, and in the neonatal period, this is one cause of a floppy baby syndrome. In the adult, a cardiopulmonary catastrophe can result in cerebellar ataxia, often with action myoclonus.

Of the metabolic causes, hypothyroidism is particularly important, because it is so easily treated. Vitamin E deficiency or a defective vitamin E transfer protein is a potentially treatable condition.

Repeated head injury, as in the "punch-drunk" syndrome, can result in ataxia, which is largely untreatable.

Chronic alcoholism may result in atrophy and degeneration of the anterior cerebellum and superior vermis resulting in an ataxia, which affects primarily the lower limbs. Apart from discontinuing the alcohol, which may prevent further damage, there is no specific treatment. Acute alcoholic intoxication causes an acute cerebellar syndrome with dysarthria, nystagmus, incoordination, and ataxia. Other intoxication that should be considered are drugs such as Dilantin, barbiturates, and lead.

Strokes involving the cerebellum occasionally present primarily as a gait problem, and posterior circulation transient ischemic attacks could present with episodic ataxia. Small vessel disease involving the brain stem or cerebellar hemispheres could ultimately present as a gait problem. Cerebellar hemorrhage is mentioned here only because it is a potentially fatal cause of unilateral ataxia and yet is eminently treatable. Sudden onset ataxia with headache or any combination of oculomotor disturbance and vertigo should always trigger an imaging study to prove or refute this possibility.

Cerebellar signs are found in about 50% of patients with multiple sclerosis, and occasionally the cerebellar syndrome is the presenting complaint. Usually, a detailed history and exquisite clinical examination demonstrate defects in other areas.

The cerebellum is an occasional site for abscess and is involved in encephalitis, particularly that of chickenpox and mumps. Children between the ages of 2 and 4 occasionally develop an acute self-limiting ataxic syndrome labeled *cerebellitis*.

In any patient presenting with a slowly progressive central neurological deficit, a brain tumor is suspect. The commonest cerebellar tumors are metastatic, followed by hemangioblastoma, glioma, and medulloblastoma. Some of these tumors have a large cystic component, and drainage of the fluid often results in restoration of normal function. Extramedullary tumors such as meningioma, vestibular schwannoma, and other posterior fossa cystic lesions, such as epidermoid cysts, may compress the brain stem or cerebellum and result in a progressive gait ataxia. Therefore, all patients with ataxia should be imaged, and most information will come from the MRI, CT scanning being subject to artifact in the posterior fossa. Systemic cancer at other sites such as the lung or ovary may cause cerebellar degeneration on an autoimmune basis.

Advances in molecular biology have resulted in new biological classifications of chronic often familial cerebellar degenerative processes previously classified as clinical syndromes on the basis of sign clusters. As the various genotypes have been defined, it has become clear that diagnosis based on the phenotype is often erroneous and of limited value, although some symptom clusters can point to specific genotypes. A single gene defect can result in a spread of signs of varying severity and distribution. Old stalwarts such as Friedreich's ataxia can usually be sorted out on the basis of pes cavus, scoliosis, absent ankle jerks with extensor plantar responses, and loss of position sense, but the syndromes are now classified as "SCA Type …" (Table 5-1). The association of epilepsy with ataxia and myoclonus, the Ramsay

Table 5-1. Molecular diagnosis of cerebellar ataxia

Name	Locus	Abnormal Protein	Repeat
SCA1	6p23	Ataxin 1	CAG
SCA2	12q24.1	Ataxin 2	CAG
SCA3	14q21	SCA3/MJDI	CAG
SCA4	16q22.1	—	—
SCA5	11	—	—
SCA6	19p13	Alpha voltage-dependent calcium channel	CAG
SCA7	3p21.1-p12	Ataxin 7	CAG
SCA8	13q21	—	CTG
SCA9	Not assigned	—	—
SCA10	22q13	SCA10	ATTCT
SCA11	15q1-q21	—	—
SCA12	5q31	Protein phosphatase 2A	CAG
SCA13	19q13	—	—
SCA14	19q13.4	—	—
SCA15	No linkage	Prion protein	—
SCA16	8q23-247.1	—	—

Hunt syndrome, is now known to be due to mitochondrial dysfunction, which can be diagnosed on muscle biopsy.

SUGGESTED READING

Bird TD. Hereditary ataxia overview. Available at www.geneclinics.org.

Brennan RW, Bergland RM. Acute cerebellar hemorrhage. Analysis and clinical findings and outcome in 12 cases. Neurology 1977;27:527.

Bronstein AM, Hood JD, Gresty MA, Panagic C. Visual control of balance in cerebellar and parkinsonian syndromes. Brain 1990;113:767.

Gilman S, Bloeldel JR, Lechtenberg R. Disorders of the Cerebellum. Philadelphia: F. A. Davis, 1981.

Hallett M, Stanhope SJ, Thomas SL, Massoquoi S. Pathophysiology of posture and gait in cerebellar ataxia. In Shimamura M, Grillner S, Edgerton VR (eds), Neurobiological Basis of Human Locomotion. Tokyo: Japan Scientific Societies Press, 1991.

Kase CS, Norrving B, Levine SR, et al. Cerebellar infarction. Clinical and anatomic observations in 66 cases. Stroke 1993;24:76.

Klockgether T, Ludtke R, Kramer B, et al. The natural history of degenerative ataxia: a retrospective study of 466 patients. Brain 1998;121:589.

C H A P T E R   S I X

Extrapyramidal Disorders

The common extrapyramidal disorders that interfere with gait share the features of slowness, akinesia,
and disequilibrium. These may be called *hypokinetic
disorders.* In contrast, hyperkinetic disorders are
characterized by excessive involuntary movement
that only occasionally interferes with gait. The patient can almost never be specific about his or her
disability and the diagnosis is made by way of a careful neurological examination.

Movement disorders arise from dysfunction in
the deep gray matter of brain, the basal ganglia. The
basal ganglia are made up of the striatum, the globus
pallidus, the substantia nigra, the subthalamic nucleus, and the thalamus. The caudate and putamen
make up the striatum. The basal ganglia project to
the cortex via the thalamus and ultimately facilitate

smooth corticospinal function so that they have a major role in motor control, tone and posture. Furthermore, they play a role in cognitive functioning.

The major input to the striatum is from the cortex (glutamate) and substantia nigra compacta (dopamine). Two output pathways from the striatum have been described, one direct and the other indirect. The direct pathway projects to the globus pallidus interna and substantia nigra reticulata (GABA, substance P, and dynorphin) and activates D1 dopamine receptors. The indirect pathway projects to the globus pallidus externa, thence to subthalamic nucleus, and then back to globus pallidus interna and substantia nigra reticulata (GABA, enkephalin) and activates D2 dopamine receptors. The projection from the globus pallidus externa to the subthalamic nucleus is inhibitory (GABA), and the projection from the subthalamic nucleus to the globus pallidus interna and substantia nigra reticulata is excitatory (glutamate).

The globus pallidus interna and substantia nigra reticulata, the output nuclei, project to the thalamus and are inhibitory (GABA). The thalamocortical pathways are excitatory (glutamate).

Corticostriatal activation of the direct pathway inhibits the globus pallidus interna and substantia nigra reticulata, which disinhibits their thalamic targets and thus facilitates thalamic excitatory projections to cortex. The net effect is a positive feed-back to cortex for the initiated movement.

Corticostriatal activation of the indirect pathway inhibits the globus pallidus externa and facilitates the subthalamic nucleus, which increases excitatory drive to the globus pallidus interna and substantia nigra reticulata. Increased output inhibits thalamic and brain stem targets. The net effect is negative feedback for movement (Figures 6-1 and 6-2).

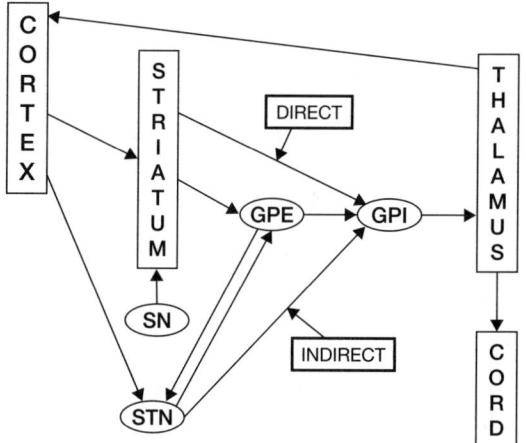

Figure 6-1. Basal ganglia connections. GPE = globus pallidus externa; GPI = globus pallidus interna; SN = substantia nigra; STN = subthalamic nucleus.

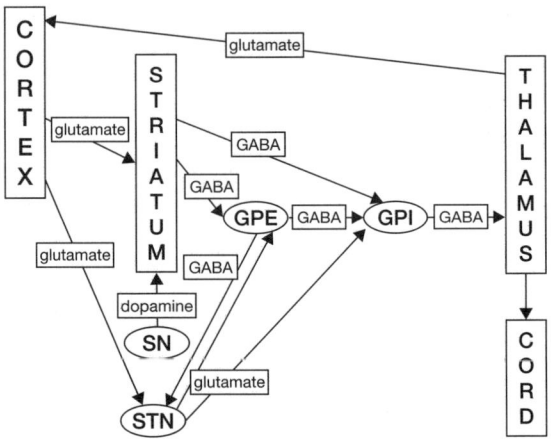

Figure 6-2. Basal ganglia connections—neurotransmitters: glutamate is excitatory, GABA is inhibitory. GPE = globus pallidus externa; GPI = globus pallidus interna; SN = substantia nigra; STN = subthalamic nucleus.

In Parkinson's disease, dopamine-producing neurons degenerate, with depigmentation and gliosis, particularly in substantia nigra compacta. The normal inhibitory dopaminergic input to D2 striatal neurons projecting to globus pallidus externa decreases. These hyperactive neurons inhibit the globus pallidus externa, whose inhibitory output to subthalamic nucleus is reduced in turn and the subthalamic nucleus becomes hyperactive. A hyperactive subthalamic nucleus increases activation of the globus pallidus interna, and this, together with decreased activation of the D1-mediated direct pathway, results in overall decreased activation of the target thalamic nuclei and their cortical projection areas.

PARKINSON'S DISEASE

Parkinson's disease is common, and its frequency increases with age. In a study of nondemented individuals in upper Manhattan, 65 years or older, the prevalence rate of Parkinson's disease was estimated at 3.2%. The disease is more common in men and less common in black populations. Recent PET studies suggest that a reduction of dopaminergic nerve terminals in the putamen by 50% is sufficient to produce clinical signs of Parkinson's disease.

First-degree relatives are 2.3 times as likely as relatives of controls to develop Parkinson's disease. Occasional families are seen with dominantly inherited Parkinson's disease and in one kindred a genetic marker on chromosome 4q21-q23 has been linked. Alpha synuclein may be the toxic substance. Certainly, Lewy bodies, a pathological hallmark finding in Parkinson's disease, stain for synuclein. A locus on chromosome 1a (Parkin gene) close to the site of the Tau gene may be important.

Smoking may protect against Parkinson's disease, and the notion of a neurotoxic cause has been bolstered by the discovery that MPTP, a synthetic street drug, can induce Parkinson's in humans and animals. A postinfective form has been recognized since the 1917 epidemic of encephalitis lethargica.

The Gait

Gait abnormalities are the presenting complaint of 12–18% of parkinsonian patients.

James Parkinson, in *An Essay on the Shaking Palsy* (1817), described the gait as follows:

> Walking becomes a task which cannot be performed without considerable attention. The legs are not raised to that height, or with that promptitude which the will directs, so that the utmost care is necessary to prevent frequent falls . . .

and

> The propensity to lean forward becomes invincible, and the patient is thereby forced to step on the toes and fore part of the feet, whilst the upper part of the body is thrown so far forward as to render it difficult to avoid falling on the face. In some cases, when this state of the malady is attained, the patient can no longer exercise himself by walking in his usual manner, but is thrown on the toes and

forepart of the feet; being, at the same time, irresistibly impelled to take much quicker and shorter steps, and thereby to adopt unwillingly a running pace. In some cases it is found necessary entirely to substitute running for walking; since otherwise the patient, on proceeding only a very few paces, would inevitably fall.

The gait is narrow based. Stride length is markedly reduced. The feet barely clear the floor. This shuffling gait is sometimes called *marche à petit pas*. The posture becomes stooped. When walking, the arms do not move but hang at the patient's side or, later, with progression of the disease, are flexed at the elbows, the hands are held in hyperpronation, flexed at the metacarpophalangeal joints, but with fingers extended and immobile. With the flexed posture the center of gravity is thrown forward, the trunk precedes the lower limbs, and the patient takes increasingly faster short steps to give the appearance of running or hurrying—a "festinating" gait. The head may become fixed in flexion.

There is a tendency to fall backward or take increasingly frequent backwards steps—"retropulsion." When asked to turn on a dime, or about-face, the patient turns with multiple small steps—"en bloc" turning. There is difficulty initiating walking, the patient takes multiple small steps on a spot before being unable to take larger strides—"start hesitation." The same phenomenon may occur as the patient walks through a doorway or has to turn— "freezing." Foot strike is often abnormal with the forefoot striking the ground before the heel.

Particularly when sitting in a soft chair, the patient may have difficulty rising. Normally one tucks the feet under the seat of the chair as one rises, so that the feet are at the center of gravity. The parkinsonian patient fails to do this and may fall back into the chair three or four times before obtaining the erect posture.

As the disease progresses there is the risk of falling. This may be due to postural instability, dyskinesias related to treatment, postural hypotension, and difficulties sitting or rising. The patient may trip over minor obstacles on the ground because each step is too small to clear.

Diagnosis

In the late stages, the diagnosis is unmistakable, but problems with diagnosis arise in the early stages of Parkinson's disease, when a mild gait disorder may be the presenting symptom. A good strategy is to observe the patient walking from the waiting room to the examining room. Apart from lack of arm swing, a narrow base and small stride length are seen. The diagnosis may be given away by the presence of hand tremor as the patient walks.

The cardinal signs of Parkinson's disease are resting tremor, bradykinesia, rigidity, and asymmetry of onset.

In addition, a host of minor signs help with the diagnosis. There is loss of facial expression, which probably results from a combination of facial bradykinesia and rigidity. There is infrequent blinking. Repeated tapping on the glabella results in persistent blinking with each tap, which does not fatigue as in normals. There is poor ocular convergence when asked to look at a close object. The skin is oily, the voice is soft, and there may be repetition of syllables within a multisyllabic word (palilalia). There may be drooling because of infrequent swallowing of saliva. The tremor becomes prominent when the patient is distracted. Muscular tone is tested by passive movement of the wrist and is increased throughout the range of movement "plastic or lead-pipe rigidity." If doubt exists, the patient is asked to rapidly tap on the knee with the contralateral hand as a distraction, which will increase the hypertonia, and if there is a superimposed tremor, a ratchet like quality to the hypertonia is produced—"cogwheel rigidity." The handwriting becomes smaller and illegible—"micrographia." Tone is increased, too, in the lower limbs, but it may be impossible to differentiate the causes of lower limb spasticity by examining the legs in isolation. If a normal person is suddenly pushed backward by pressure to the chest when standing, an immediate contraction occurs in the muscles necessary to maintain equilibrium. The parkinsonian patient is set in motion by a feeble push and may stagger backward.

Rarely, the signs seem concentrated in the lower limbs, so-called "lower-half Parkinson's." Lower-body parkinsonism is often correlated with multiple small strokes. As such, these patients are more likely to have, in addition to the extrapyramidal signs of Parkinson's disease, corticospinal signs, incontinence, and pseudobulbar affect.

If the signs are particularly subtle, yet clearly present, and the symptoms upsetting, it may be worth a clinical trial of antiparkinsonian medication—improvement will support the diagnosis.

Patients with postural instability and gait difficulty (PIGD) are older, are more likely to be cognitively impaired, and have a more rapidly progressive course than patients with tremor-dominant Parkinson's disease.

PARKINSON PLUS SYNDROMES

Although about 75% of patients with hypokinetic extrapyramidal syndromes have true Parkinson's disease, other degenerative disorders have, as part of their clinical cluster of signs, extrapyramidal signs of the parkinsonian type. None of them respond very well to L-dopa replacement therapy and failure to respond to symptomatic treatment should at least arouse suspicion for one of these conditions.

Multiple System Atrophy

Multiple system atrophy is a term used to encompass patients with overlapping features of autonomic failure (Shy-Drager syndrome), striatonigral degeneration, and sporadic olivopontocerebellar atrophy. Clinically, these patients show parkinsonian features to a greater or lesser extent together with autonomic dysfunction and cerebellar ataxia in any combination. Some may have pyramidal signs in the legs. Two thirds of patients with multiple system atrophy show some response to L-dopa, at least early on, so that the diagnosis is often delayed.

Progressive Supranuclear Palsy

Progressive supranuclear palsy (Steele-Richardson-Olszewski syndrome) should be considered in patients with progressive parkinsonism and supranuclear disturbances of ocular motility. These patients present particularly with disturbances of gait and balance and frequent falls, so that falling early in the course of illness is a clue to the diagnosis. The gait is characterized by a broad base and a tendency to have the knees and trunk extended and the arms slightly abducted. Some patients show freezing, micrographia, hypophonia, and blepharospasm. Falling is caused by uncompensated loss of postural reflexes and freezing especially on turns.

The term *supranuclear gaze palsy* refers to dysfunction of upper motor neuron control of eye movements, the earliest sign of which is paresis of voluntary down gaze. The defect can be overcome by oculocephalic maneuvers (doll's eye testing), proving that the third nerves or lower motor neuron pathway is intact, but some patients lose this feature late in the disease, suggesting nuclear involvement. Dystonia may take the form of blepharospasm and occasionally patients have apraxia of eyelid opening or closing. Pseudobulbar signs may be present with emotional lability, dysarthria, and spastic ataxic monotonous low-pitched dysarthria with stuttering or palilalia. A mild subcortical dementia can ensue.

Corticobasal Ganglionic Degeneration

Asymmetry in a complex neurodegenerative syndrome with some parkinsonian features should suggest the diagnosis of corticobasal ganglionic degeneration. Limb dystonia, ideomotor apraxia, myoclonus, and an akinetic-rigid syndrome with late-onset gait or balance problems were found to be the best predictors of the syndrome in 10 autopsy-proven cases. Focal rigidity and dystonia with contractures, rest and action tremor, cortical sensory loss with an "alien hand" phenomenon, and late dementia as well as impaired convergence and vertical gaze palsies and extensor plantar reflexes complete the clinical syndrome.

There is an overlap in clinical and pathological features between corticobasal ganglionic degeneration, progressive supranuclear palsy, and Pick's disease—in the last, predominant frontal lobe and language dysfunction with relatively preserved memory, at least early on, provide the clue.

Diffuse Lewy Body Disease

An overlap syndrome comprising some features of Alzheimer's disease and some features of Parkinson's disease is now recognized to be the second most common cause of degenerative dementia in the elderly. Prominent visual hallucinations with fluctuating attention and motor signs of Parkinson's disease suggest the diagnosis. The case may be strengthened by the finding of myoclonus, lack of rest tremor, and as in virtually all of the Parkinson plus syndromes, lack of response to levodopa.

SECONDARY PARKINSONISM

The presence of an extrapyramidal syndrome of the parkinsonian type should arouse some thought of symptomatic rather than idiopathic parkinsonism. Following the influenza epidemic of 1917, there was a fallout of postencephalitic parkinsonism, which had the additional features of oculogyric crises, blepharospasm, tics, and other movement disorders.

Perhaps of more current relevance is the syndrome of drug-induced parkinsonism, because it may be reversible on withdrawal of the offending drug. The major causes are the neuroleptics, and two thirds of patients will recover within 7 weeks of withdrawal. It is possible that some patients may have an underlying subclinical Parkinson's disease aggravated by the drugs. Other drugs on the list include dopa-depleting drugs such as reserpine, and occasionally extrapyramidal signs are produced as side effects of lithium, flunarizine, or cinnarizine.

Delayed-onset parkinsonism is sometimes seen after severe anoxia, trauma, or carbon monoxide intoxication.

Chronic exposure to manganese can induce the parkinsonian syndrome, often with neuropsychiatric symptoms and an action rather than a rest tremor, with cerebellar signs.

Rarely, parkinsonian signs are secondary to hypoparathyroidism, chronic liver failure, and mitochondrial encephalopathies.

ORTHOSTATIC TREMOR

Patients complain of tremulousness or shakiness when standing; they may fall unless they sit or walk; then the tremor may disappear entirely. It can be induced by pressing the feet against the foot of the bed while supine. Electrophysiological recordings define a fast tremor (14–18 Hz) in the lower limbs as well as in the upper limbs. These patients respond to clonazepam and not beta blockers or alcohol.

SUGGESTED READING

Calne DB, Chu N-S, Huan CC, et al. Manganism and idiopathic parkinsonism: similarities and differences. Neurology 1994;44:1583.

Cummings JL. Depression and Parkinson's disease: a review. Am J Psychiatry 1992;149:443.

Feany MB, Dickson DW. Neurodegenerative disorders with extensive tau pathology: a comparative study and review. Ann Neurol 1996;40:139.

Fitzgerald PM, Jankovic J. Lower body parkinsonism: evidence for a vascular etiology. Mov Disord 1989; 4:249.

Fitzgerald PM, Jankovic J. Orthostatic tremor: an association with essential tremor. Mov Disord 1991;6:60.

Goedert M, Spillantini MG, Sexpell LL, et al. From genetics to pathology: tau and alpha-synuclein assemblies in neurodegenerative disease. Philos Trans R Soc Lond B Biol Sci 2001;356:213.

Graybiel AM, Aosaki T, Flaherty AW, et al. The basal ganglia and adaptive motor control. Science 1994; 265:1826.

Jankovic J. Parkinsonian syndromes. In Kurlan R (ed), Treatment of Movement Disorders. Philadelphia: J. B. Lippincott, 1995:95.

Krusz JC, Koller WC, Ziegler DK. Historical review: abnormal movements associated with epidemic encephalitis lethargica. Mov Disord 1987;2:137.

Langston JW, Ballard PA, Tetrud JW, et al. Chronic parkinsonism in humans due to a product of meperidine analogue synthesis. Science 1983; 219:979.

Levy R, Hazrati LN, Herrero MT, et al. Reevaluation of the functional anatomy of the basal ganglia in normal and parkinsonian states. Neuroscience 1997; 76:335.

Litvan I, Agid Y, Goetz C, et al. Accuracy of the clinical diagnosis of corticobasal degeneration: a clinicopathological study. Neurology 1997;48:119.

Litvan I, Campbell G, Mangone CA, et al. Which clinical features differentiate progressive supranuclear palsy (Steele-Richardson-Olszewski syndrome) from related disorders? A clinicopathological study. Brain 1997;120:65a.

McKeith IG, Galasko D, Kosaka K, et al. Consensus guidelines for the clinical and pathological diagnosis of dementia with Lewy bodies (DLB): report of the conostium on DLB international workshop. Neurology 1996;47:113.

Obeso JA, Rodriguez MC, DeLong MR. Basal ganglia pathophysiology: a critical revue. Adv Neurol 1997; 74:3.

Rebeiz JJ, Kolodny EH, Richardson EP. Corticodentato-nigral degeneration with neuronal achromatasia. Arch Neurol 1968;18:20.

Steele JC, Richardson JC, Olszewski J. Progressive supranuclear palsy: a heterogenous degeneration involving the brain stem, basal ganglia and cerebellum with vertical gaze and pseudobulbar palsy, nuchal dystonia and dementia. Arch Neurol 1964;10:333.

Tanner CM, Langston JW. Do environmental toxins cause Parkinson's disease? A critical review. Neurology 1990;S3:17.

Wenning GK, Tison F, Shlomo BY, et al. Multiple system atrophy: a review of 203 pathologically proven cases. Mov Disord 1997;12:133.

Frontal Lobe Dysfunction

The highest centers for the control of walking are in the frontal lobe.

The decision to walk is initiated in the frontal lobes, and after gait ignition, coordination and control of walking depends on an interplay and complex feedback system involving proprioception, cerebellar function, and basal ganglia function as well as motor output. Frontal lobe dysfunction may result in isolated gait ignition failure, the more common "frontal gait disorder" and "frontal ataxia."

Some use the term *apraxia of gait* for frontal gait disorder. *Apraxia* may not be the best label. The term *apraxia* is usually defined as the inability to perform a learned motor act in the presence of intact subcortical mechanisms. The objection to the use of this term in the context of gait abnormalities is that gait is not a "learned motor act," rather it is an inherent function of the nervous system and, in animals at least, present at birth. In humans, gait develops naturally with normal maturation of the nervous system.

Bruns in 1892 coined the term *frontal ataxia* because of the severe disequilibrium; and Van Bogaert and Martin, in 1929, suggested that frontal gait ataxia might result from a disconnection between the idea of walking and the motor programs required to walk. Their patient had a frontal abscess, walked with small steps, her legs became tangled, and she was unable to make purposeful movements of the legs on command but could do so spontaneously.

THE GAIT

Ignition Failure

The patient cannot initiate or sustain normal walking. At initiation, the patient hesitates, may take three or four steps on the spot, the feet barely clearing the floor, and then steps forward on a narrow base. Stride length is markedly shortened, and with ambulation, the feet barely clear the floor to give the impression of shuffling. Freezing, a sudden halt in leg movement, sometimes occurs. Curiously, once the patient gets under way, the stride lengthens and foot clearance normalizes. Postural responses are normal and falls are rare. The majority of patients show no associated neurological signs, and brain imaging is normal. Some patients go on to develop a frontal lobe syndrome with a more classic frontal gait disorder, suggesting a progressive underlying pathology.

Frontal Ataxia

There is a breakdown of leg movements required for ambulation. The feet may cross or move in a direction inappropriate to the center of gravity, so that the gait looks bizarre.

Frontal Gait Disorder

There may be difficulty with initiation as in patients with pure ignition failure. Movement freezes, the base is usually narrow, the stride length is shortened and shuffling. The patient shows hesitation on turns. Frontal gait disorder differs from ignition failure in that there is disequilibrium, impaired ongoing locomotion, and frequently other signs of frontal lobe dysfunction. With progression, there are impaired righting reactions and loss of protective reflexes, so that falls are common.

THE SIGNS

The signs of frontal lobe dysfunction, apart from the gait disorder, may be divided into those relating to cognitive loss and elementary signs. In general, the term *frontal lobe syndrome* implies dysfunction of the prefrontal cortex. Mesulam has characterized the prefrontal cortex as the site for the confluence of two functional axes: one for working memory, executive function, and attention and another for comportment (conduct). Frontal lobe dysfunction can result in two broad syndromes. One is characterized by slowness of thought, loss of initiative, loss of creativity with apathy, and emotional blunting—frontal abulia. The other has impulsivity and loss of judgment and insight—frontal disinhibition. Lesions in the orbitofrontal and medial frontal areas are likely to cause disinhibition, whereas dorso lateral frontal lobe dysfunction is more likely to cause the abulic syndrome.

Cognitive Signs

Simple bedside mental status tests may show the patient to be completely normal, but one can frequently tease out signs of frontal dysfunction. Attention and concentration, the ability to maintain a coherent stream of thought, and verbal fluency and memory retrieval are easily and quickly tested. The lack of mental flexibility or poor attentional mechanisms may interfere with the ability to reverse the days of the week, or months of the year, or count forwards in threes. Word generation can be tested by asking the patient to name as many words as possible beginning with the letters F, A, and S—allocation of 1 minute for each letter should generate 36–40 words over 3 minutes.

The patient may be unable to resist immediate but inappropriate responses and have difficulty programming selected sequential responses. The "go/no-go" paradigm tests the former, and the motor sequencing task (often called the *Luria sequencing task*) tests the latter.

To perform the go/no-go test, with the hand palm down on a flat surface, the patient is asked to quickly raise and immediately lower the index finger in response to a single tap of a pencil (go), and produce no response if the examiner taps twice in rapid succession (no-go).

In the Luria motor sequencing test, one demonstrates for the patient and then asks for a series of repeats of three hand postures—striking a tabletop with a clenched fist, and open palm, and then the edge of the hand.

Occasionally imitative or stimulus bound behavior is seen. The patient shows a remarkable tendency to imitate to the examiner's gestures and behaviors, even when no instruction to do so has been given. The balance between the parietal function, oriented toward extrapersonal events, and frontal function, oriented toward internal mental processes, is disturbed in favor of the former. (The opposite would be the neglect seen in parietal lobe lesions.)

Judgment is usually considered to be part of comportment. It is virtually impossible to test this in the office or at the bedside by constructing an artificial situation and asking the patient to react. Judgment can be tested only by real-life observation. The patient may act recklessly when faced with the real situation yet give perfect answers to hypothetical problems.

Elementary Signs

The elementary signs include paratonia, grasp and pull reflexes, and palmomental reflexes. These primitive reflexes emerge when the lesion extends posteriorly into the motor and premotor areas of frontal lobe.

Paratonia (gegenhalten). When attempting to passively test the tone of the limbs, one detects a variable irregular waxing and waning of tone of the major muscle groups, almost as if the patient is attempting to help or hinder the examiner.

Grasp reflex. Stimulation of the palm of hand results in an automatic grasp, so firm that it may be difficult for the examiner to withdraw his or her fingers.

Pull reflex. If one hooks one's fingers under the patient's semiflexed fingers, a strong flexion contraction of the fingers results.

Palmomental reflex. Scratching the palm of hand results in a twitch of the facial muscles below the lip on the ipsilateral side.

In patients with severe advanced frontal dementia it may be possible to elicit a suck and rooting reflex, as is present in neonates.

In general, in patients with gait disorders arising from pathology in the frontal lobe, if cognitive impairment is present, the abulic syndrome is to be expected.

PATHOLOGY

The likely candidates for pathology in patients presenting with a frontal gait disorder, with abulia, include

1. Subcortical arteriosclerotic encephalopathy and the lacunar state (Binswanger's disease). Marche à petit pas, a short-stepped military

gait with an upright trunk posture and stiff legs has been called *lower-half parkinsonism* or *arteriosclerotic parkinsonism* and is associated particularly with vascular disease in the frontal lobes. The pathology includes multiple lacunes and demyelination, particularly around the frontal horns, with an MRI picture of high T-2 signal capping the ventricles.

2. Hydrocephalus.
3. Degenerative atrophy.

Space-taking lesions are immediately discovered when the patient is imaged and present no diagnostic problem.

NORMAL PRESSURE HYDROCEPHALUS

Ventriculomegaly in the elderly is usually due to atrophy. If the cortical ribbon is atrophic and the sulci enlarged, a degenerative disorder is likely. In normal pressure hydrocephalus (NPH), the ventricles are enlarged out of proportion to cortical atrophy.

NPH as a clinical syndrome was first described by Adams, Fisher, Hakim, and colleagues in 1965. They treated three patients with communicating hydrocephalus and the cerebrospinal fluid (CSF) was under normal pressure. Unexpectedly, the patients improved with repeated spinal taps or a shunt procedure. Nevertheless, the issue of so-called normal pressure hydrocephalus has aroused some skepticism, probably because of overdiagnosis and misdiagnosis. In this admittedly rare syndrome, although the ventricles are enlarged, random ventricular pressure readings may be normal, hence, the label. Pressures can usually be shown to be intermittently raised, so that a better name for the complex would be *intermittent normal pressure hydrocephalus.*

Even though often considered a cause of gait disorder in the elderly, normal pressure hydrocephalus is a difficult diagnosis to prove, although enlarged frontal horns are correlated with gait disorders. Yakovlev suggested that the fibers from the leg area are stretched as they course around the dilated lateral ventricles, and Fisher related the span of the anterior horns to the degree of gait abnormality.

Pathogenesis

A good deal of epidemiological evidence links hypertension and communicating hydrocephalus. The mechanism is unclear but there may be failure of CSF absorption in the face of increased superior sagittal sinus venous pressure together with increased intraventricular pulse pressure from the choroid plexus. It remains to be shown whether hypertension causes hydrocephalus, hydrocephalus causes hypertension, or perhaps they cause each other.

In communicating hydrocephalus, there is an obstruction to CSF flow outside the ventricular system. This may be a complication of traumatic or spontaneous subarachnoid hemorrhage or of meningitis, where the meningeal process partially blocks CSF pathways acutely or insidiously. Often no specific cause can be found.

In noncommunicating hydrocephalus the relative obstruction is within the ventricular system. Blockage may be caused by a tumor, such as a colloid cyst of the third ventricle, or aqueduct stenosis. Here, too, the pressure may be normal at times.

Intracranial pressure is high in the early stages of hydrocephalus, but once the ventricles dilate, they are maintained in their distended state at a lower or normal pressure. Pascal's law states that the force on the walls of a hollow container is equal to the product of the pressure of the fluid and the area of the wall ($F = P \times A$). In the ventricular system, the force on the walls of the ventricles should be equal to the product of the cerebrospinal fluid pressure and the ventricular area. A bicycle tire carries a pressure of around 30 pounds, whereas the much larger tire of a huge tractor is maintained inflated at a much lower pressure. As the ventricles increase in size, a much lower pressure keeps them distended.

The Gait in NPH

Disturbance of gait is usually the first sign and considered the most important symptom—decreased gait velocity, reduced stride length, and reduced step height during the swing phase of the gait cycle. The gait is somewhat broad based with the feet rotated outward. Gait-associated movements of arm swing are unimpaired. The normal variability of step width and foot angles is decreased, leading to an insufficient compensation of body sway required to avoid obstacles in the path—decreased dynamic equilibrium. After shunting or spinal tap, gait velocity increases by about 20%.

Both NPH and Parkinson's disease share a hypokinetic gait, which includes short steps, leg rigidity, flexed posture, and impaired postural reflexes. An enlarged step width and increased foot angles are almost never seen in Parkinson's disease, whereas in NPH, a widened step width or larger foot angles are commonly present. While visual and acoustic cues can improve the gait in Parkinson's disease, they do not affect the gait in NPH.

Diagnosis

The clinical triad of frontal cognitive loss, gait disorder, and urinary incontinence suggests the diagnosis of NPH. Yet, only 50% of patients with the classical triad improve with surgery, and shunt surgery has a long-term complication rate of approximately 30%. Perhaps, the explanation for the failure rate is a diverse etiology of the signs and symptoms. Certainly, none of the presenting signs is specific for hydrocephalus. Furthermore, even in those who respond favorably, the gait and incontinence usually improve but cognition improves in only 50% of patients. Therefore, initial enthusiasm for shunting waned when patients did not respond and further efforts were made to confirm the diagnosis and exclude from shunting those patients who simply had cerebral atrophy.

On the clinical side, a history of dementia for more than 2 years predicts a poor response to shunting. If the gait abnormality began before or at the same time as a dementia, the chances for a successful surgical outcome are increased. If there is a secondary cause of hydrocephalus, such as subarachnoid hemorrhage, meningitis, head injury, or brain surgery, the chances of improvement with shunting are increased. Conversely, a history of alcohol abuse is a poor prognostic indicator for surgical success, as is the presence of aphasia.

Over the years, various tests to prove the diagnosis and select patients for shunting have been suggested; only a few have stood the test of time.

Investigations Designed to Prove Normal Pressure Hydrocephalus

Imaging studies. Computed tomography (CT) shows ventricular enlargement out of proportion to cerebral atrophy. Hippocampal atrophy suggests Alzheimer's disease, but periventricular lucencies suggestive of ischemic pathology do not preclude clinical improvement after a shunt.

Magnetic resonance imaging (MRI) is particularly sensitive to white matter lesions and lends itself to volumetric evaluation of the hippocampus, which is not atrophic in NPH. T-2 images may show a flow void sign in the aqueduct, which correlates with the velocity of pulsatile CSF flow. In shunt-responsive communicating hydrocephalus, aqueduct flow velocity may be increased, but successful shunting does not necessarily result in a decrease of the CSF flow void sign.

Regional cerebral blood flow studies. Regional cerebral blood flow is decreased in the parietotemporal areas in Alzheimer's disease. Conversely, it is decreased in the frontal areas in hydrocephalus. The calculated ratio of frontal to posterior regional blood flow is a reasonably good indicator of the likelihood of success with shunting—a low ratio predicts a symptomatic hydrocephalus and a high ratio predicts a pseudosymptomatic hydrocephalus in patients with Alzheimer's disease.

Removal of CSF. Lumbar puncture with removal of about 40 cc of CSF may be followed by transient or, in some cases prolonged, clinical improvement. There is a high rate of false negative results, and the predictive accuracy is therefore limited. This test is now used worldwide, probably because it is easy, rapid, and cheap; and a strikingly positive result usually suggests that a shunt will work.

Cisternography. Radioisotope cisternography, although formerly a popular test, is unreliable and does not add to the diagnostic accuracy of combined clinical and imaging criteria.

Pressure monitoring. Continuous intracranial pressure monitoring may show increased pressure waves with a frequency of 0.5–2 per minute (B-waves). B-waves are present in healthy people but can exceed 50% of observation time in NPH.

Hydrodynamic tests. Infusion of sterile normal saline or artificial CSF into the subarachnoid space at time of lumbar puncture measures CSF absorption mechanisms. In patients with normal absorption, infusion at a rate approximately twice the usual rate of CSF formation results in a modestly predictable CSF pressure elevation. In communicating hydrocephalus, the capacity to absorb this additional fluid is reduced and, with infusion, the CSF pressure rises abruptly. A three-way stopcock permits measurement of pressure with a simple displacement manometer. Prolonged infusion at a rate of 0.76 ml per minute corresponds to twice the rate of absorption. The resistance to CSF outflow can be measured via the lumbar rout, or via a ventricular catheter. CSF reabsorption can be estimated by a constant lumboventricular or ventriculoventricular CSF infusion at different CSF pressures.

The diagnostic accuracy of these tests is operator dependent but some authors report very reliable results.

With a short history, a known cause of hydrocephalus, predominance of gait disorder, and imaging suggesting hydrodynamic hydrocephalus, about 50–70% of patients do well after surgery. It is certainly justified to shunt patients with an unequivocally positive CSF tap test. Certain surgeons also perform hydrodynamic tests. However, the commonest cause of the clinical triad of dementia, gait disorder, and incontinence remains subcortical arteriosclerotic encephalopathy.

SUGGESTED READING

Adams RD, Fisher CM, Hakim MD, et al. Symptomatic occult hydrocephalus with "normal" cerebrospinal fluid pressure. N Engl J Med 1965;273:117.

Black PM. Idiopathic normal-pressure hydrocephalus. Results of shunting in 62 patients. J Neurosurg 1980;52:371.

Borgesen SE, Gjerris F, Sorensen SC. Intracranial pressure and conductance to outflow of cerebrospinal fluid in normal-pressure hydrocephalus. J Neurosurg 1979;50:489.

Fisher CM. Hydrocephalus as a cause of disturbances of gait in the elderly. Neurology 1982;32:1358.

Katzman R, Hussey F. A simple constant infusion manometric test for measurement of CSF absorption. Neurology 1970;20:534.

Lyons MK, Meyer FB. Cerebrospinal fluid physiology and the management of increased intracranial pressure. Mayo Clin Proc 1990;65:684.

Nitz WR, Bradley Jr, WG, Watanabe AS, et al. Flow dynamics of cerebrospinal fluid: assessment with phase-contrast velocity MR imaging performed with retrospective cardiac gating. Radiology 1992; 183:395.

Stolze H, Kuhtz-Buschbeck JP, Drucke H, et al. Comparative analysis of the gait disorder of normal pressure hydrocephalus and Parkinson's disease. J Neurol Neurosurg Psychiatry 2001;70:289–297.

Wikkelso C, Andersson H, Blomstrand C, Lindqvist G. The clinical effects of lumbar puncture in normal pressure hydrocephalus. J Neurol Neurosurg Psychiatry 1982;45:64.

Yakovlev PI. Paraplegias of hydrocephalies. Am J Ment Def 1947;51:561.

CHAPTER EIGHT

Psychogenic Factors in Gait Disorders

Patients with old age gait disorder are frequently fearful of falling. At times, fear aggravates a minor dysfunction or inhibits normal gait. It is possible to separate patients whose main disability has been termed *cautious gait* or simply *fear of falling* from those whose disability is grossly psychiatric in origin.

CAUTIOUS GAIT

The classic description was provided by Murray, Kory, and Clarkson in 1969:

> The walking performance of older men gave the impression of a guarded or restrained type of walking in an attempt to obtain maximum stability and security. The walking of older men resembled that of someone walking on a slippery surface.

In normal elderly subjects, an increase in foot-floor clearance during the early swing phase of gait provides additional security against tripping. Other adaptations to provide safer gait in the elderly include a reduction in stride length, increased stance time, and double support time. The elderly show a tendency toward a stooped posture, reduced stride, and loss of the normal heel-to-toe sequence of foot-floor contact. There is no akinesia in normal aging.

An exaggeration of this gait, often with the conscious awareness of the need for caution to adjust for imbalance and avoid falls, called the *cautious gait* by Nutt, Marsden, and Thompson, was regarded as a compensatory adaptation with an appropriate response to real or perceived disequilibrium. The adaptation is the salient characteristic; and the precipitant ranges from a mechanically insecure base, as in walking up or down stairs or on a slippery surface, through the subtle manifestation of any of the causes of gait disorder discussed in this book associated with anxiety.

FEAR OF FALLING

Fear of falling is strongly associated with a history of recent falls and is present in about 50% of patients who have fallen. Higher levels of fear of falling and hurting oneself in the next year are associated with higher levels of physical dysfunction, and the fear itself is related to a lower quality of life; timid, preoccupied patients limit their activities. While the fear may be exaggerated, it often has a rational basis and too little caution could be detrimental. Given a rational basis, comorbidities found in patients with fear of falling include virtually all causes of gait disorder in the elderly.

Initially, fear of falling produces a patient who is appropriately more alert to potential hazards in the environment, but it may progress to disabling fear in specific situations resulting in avoidance behaviors. So severe may be the anxiety that it qualifies as a phobia—patients with fear of falling in open spaces where there is no visuospatial support may resort to crawling on hands and knees and this may culminate in a wheelchair existence.

In one study, fear of falling was associated with increased mortality. One third of patients with postfall syndrome died within 4 months of hospital admission due to pulmonary embolism, myocardial infarction, or bronchopneumonia.

Fear of falling may be more frequent in women.

DEPRESSION

Severely depressed patients may develop psychomotor retardation, with slowness of all movements and abnormal hypokinetic gait. Depressed patients walk with a lifting motion of the leg and reduced stride length, whereas normal control subjects propel themselves forward.

PSYCHOGENIC GAIT DISORDER

Abasia-astasia is the inability to stand or walk in the absence of other neurological abnormalities, so named by Jaccoud, Charcot, and Blocq in 1888. Camptocormia is characterized by exaggerated trunk flexion of functional etiology. Some psychiatrists have attempted to distinguish a phobic from an hysterical form of the disorder.

Abasia-astasia is a fairly gross presentation of hysteria and not at all subtle. The substrate of gross hysteria like this includes children, unsophisticated patients, and occasionally a patient with limbic epilepsy. Many of Charcot's patients were rural, simple people who moved to Paris. The prognosis in children and adolescents is good—in one series of 27 patients with abasia-astasia, 22 were in good health 5–22 years later, although 9 had minor complaints. In adults, symptom substitution can be a problem.

Lempert, Brandt, Dieterich, and Huppert analyzed the clinical characteristics of psychogenic gait disorder from videotapes and suggested six characteristic features that support the diagnosis of psychogenesis. They occurred alone or in combination in 97% of their patients:

1. Momentary fluctuations of stance and gait, often in response to suggestion.
2. Excessive slowness or hesitation of locomotion incompatible with neurological disease.
3. "Psychogenic" result from a Romberg test, with a build-up of swaying amplitudes after a silent latency or with improvement by distraction.
4. Uneconomic postures with wastage of muscular energy.
5. "Walking on ice," characterized by small cautious steps with fixed ankle joints.
6. Sudden buckling of the knees, usually without falls.

The quintessential prototypes of a hysterical gait disorder are either excessive slowness and stiffness or maintenance of postural control on narrow base with flailing arms and excessive trunk sway without falling (tightrope walking). Simulated weakness in one or both legs, ataxia, and trembling are other manifestations; and normal neurological function (apart from the gait) must be demonstrated. The experienced clinician is usually fairly confident of the diagnosis, but normal imaging studies and a dramatic cure with appropriate psychotherapy is the best diagnostic evidence.

CONFUSIONAL STATES

Although in the inpatient hospital setting, one seldom gets the confused patient out of bed to test gait, these patients frequently have a gait disorder. Because the commonest cause of confusion is a metabolic or toxic encephalopathy, asterixis and polymyoclonia are often present; when these affect the lower limbs when the patient is standing or walking, they may cause falls or an unsteady gait. Even without an associated movement disorder, these patients sometimes have a wondering or broad-based gait, probably on the basis of decreased attentional mechanisms, the hallmark of a confusional state.

SOCIOCULTURAL DIFFERENCES IN GAIT

People from different social environments have different gait velocities. One study measured gait velocities in Berlin, Germany, and compared them to subjects living in the Tyrol, a rural setting. Healthy subjects in Berlin showed faster gait velocity than their counterparts in Tyrol, and this difference extended even to patients with Parkinson's disease.

SUGGESTED READING

Arfken CL, Lach HW, Birge SJ, Miller JP. The prevalence and correlates of fear of falling in elderly persons living in the community. Am J Public Health 1994; 84:565.

Bhala RP, O'Donnell J, Thoppil E. Phobic fear of falling and its clinical management. Phys Ther 1982;62:187.

Ebersbach G, Sojer M, Muller J, et al. Sociocultural differences in gait. Mov Disorders 2000;15:1145.

Elble RJ, Hughes L, Higgens C. The syndrome of senile gait. J Neurol 1992;239:71.

Jette A, Assmann S, Peterson EW. Fear of falling and activity restriction: the survey of activities and fear of falling in the elderly (SAFE). J Gerontol B Psychol Sci Soc Sci 1998;53:43–50.

Keane JR. Hysterical gait disorders: 60 cases. Neurology 1989;39:586.

Lawrence RH, Tennstedt SL, Kasten LE, et al. Intensity and correlates of fear of falling and hurting oneself in the next year: baseline findings from a Roybal Center fear of falling intervention. J Aging Health 1998;10:267.

Lempert T, Brandt T, Dieterich M, Huppert D. How to identify psychogenic disorders of stance and gait. A video study in 37 patients. J Neurol 1991;238:140.

Marks I, Bebbington P. Space phobia: syndrome or agorophobic variant. Med J 1976;2:345.

Murray MP, Kory RC, Clarkson BH. Walking patterns in healthy old men. J Gerontol 1969;24:169.

Nutt JG, Marsden CD, Thompson MD. Human walking and higher-level gait disorders, particularly in the elderly. Neurology 1993;43:268.

Sloman L, Berridge M, Homatidis S, et al. Gait patterns of depressed patients and normal subjects. Am J Psychiatry 1982;139:94.

Stickler GB, Cheung-Patton A. Astasia abasia. A conversion reaction. Prognosis. Clin Pediatr [Philadelphia] 1989;28:12.

Walker JE, Howland J. Falls and fear of falling among elderly persons living in the community: occupational therapy interventions. Am J Occup Ther 1991;45:119.

Nonneurologic Causes of Gait Disorders in the Elderly

Although nonneurologic disorders can independently cause significant dysfunction, gait disorders are frequently of multifactorial origin, and an interplay of neurologic impairment and nonneurologic problems may result in a gait disorder sufficient to impair mobility and precipitate falls.

The nonneurologic causes of gait disorders are best considered in terms of site or organ specificity (Table 9-1), but more than one abnormality can be present in the same patient at the same time. A complete evaluation of the patient with gait disorder, therefore, requires not only an exquisitely detailed neurologic examination but also a detailed general medical examination.

Table 9-1. Nonneurologic causes of gait disorder

Foot
  Orthopedic deformities
  Callus and corn
  Interdigital neuroma
  Plantar fasciitis
  Metatarsal joint osteoarthritis and synovitis
Ankle
  Arthritis
  Achilles tendonitis and tendon rupture
  Ruptured posterior tibial tendon
Knee
  Arthritis
  Lax ligaments
  Cartilage pathology
Hip
  Arthritis
  Impacted fracture
  Trochanteric bursitis
Spine
  Osteoporosis
  Metastatic deposits
  Spinal claudication
  Disc degeneration and osteoarthritis
Vascular and Respiratory
  Vascular claudication
  Angina
  Heart failure
  Respiratory failure
  Arrhythmia
  Postural hypotension

Table 9-1. *(continued)*

Drugs
  Sedatives of all kinds
  Diuretics
  Hypotensive agents
  Psychotropic agents
  Cardiac drugs—nitrates, procainamide,
    beta-blockers
  Alcohol
Visual Failure
  Glaucoma
  Cataracts
  Macular degeneration
  Field cut
  Diplopia

As always, evaluation begins with the history. Whereas patients with pure neurologic dysfunction rarely can pinpoint the cause of the problem, patients with nonneurologic causes of gait disorder frequently indicate the source of the problem, be it pain, visual dysfunction, or dyspnea.

The nonneurologic causes of gait disorder are considered in ascending fashion, with a review of abnormalities of the feet and ankles, more proximal joints, lumbar spine, cardiorespiratory difficulties, and finally the role of vision in gait.

THE FEET

Foot physiology has been studied in detail. During barefoot standing, peak pressures under the heel are 2.6 times greater than under the forefoot, and the plantar surface of the heel supports 60.5% of body weight, whereas the forefoot supports 28.1%, the mid foot 7.8%, and the toes 3.6%.

The gait cycle consists of a swing phase and a stance phase, the former occupies 62% of time and the latter 38%. In normal walking, the sequence of events is heel-strike to foot-flat, then foot-flat to heel-off, and then to toe-off. Control of foot and ankle joint movement is mainly via the dorsiflexors and plantar flexors of the ankle and to some extent by the intrinsic muscles of the feet. During normal gait, the center of pressure moves rapidly from the heel to the metatarsal head area, then on to the great toe. Another peak of pressure under the forefoot occurs during heel-rise and toe-off.

With normal aging, stride and step length decrease and the swing phase occupies less time. There is decreased out-toeing and decreased ankle plantar flexion after heel-strike during fast walking.

Normal foot function may be hindered by orthopedic deformities or painful conditions of the foot. Orthopedic deformities include varus or valgus alignment, pes cavus, or simply hammer toes. These abnormalities are evident on simple inspection.

Elucidation by history or by examination of those factors that aggravate or trigger pain gives the clue to the cause. Thus, pain in the metatarsal area on standing or walking suggests local pathology that may be as simple as a painful corn or callus. The finding of local tenderness if pressure is applied to the plantar aspect of the metatarsal heads, together with tenderness on side-to-side compression of the distal foot suggests the presence of an interdigital neuroma. Pain in the sole during the initial steps from a resting position suggests plantar fasciitis, which may be confirmed by the finding of local tenderness to pressure, increased with the toes held dorsiflexed. Because of the tenderness, patients shift weight to other areas of the foot, and the abnormal gait in itself evokes pain remote from the plantar fascia. Osteoarthritis of the first metatarsophalangeal joint is common, diagnosed by the finding of spurring, limited painful movement, and tenderness of the joint. Synovitis of the lesser metatarsophalangeal joints is diagnosed by finding swelling of the joint and toe with discrete tenderness and fullness and the patient complains of pain induced by dorsiflexion of the joint during heel-rise. Local tenderness of the metatarsals to pressure might suggest a stress fracture.

THE MORE PROXIMAL JOINTS

Degenerative arthritis of the ankle joint restricts the flexion required during the foot-flat part of stance and results in the decreased stride length. This may be associated with irritation or erosion of the Achilles tendon by posterior calcaneal spurs causing local pain. Rupture of the posterior tibial tendon results in acquired flatfoot, and gait is impaired by pain and limitation of heel-rise.

Arthritis of the knee results in a stiff-legged gait, with the knee partially flexed and often inwardly rotated. Lax knee joint tendons allow for lateral bowing of the knee as weight is taken. Examination of the knee will demonstrate crepitation on passive movement, sometimes an associated effusion and positive patellar tap sign, and lax ligaments.

Hip joint arthritis presents with pain on walking and restricts movement at the hip on the affected side, resulting in a characteristic limp. With normal walking, the body's center of gravity shifts away from the foot touching the ground. With hip disease, there is a tendency to displace the body over the painful hip, which can be alleviated if a cane is carried on the uninvolved side—this shortens the duration of weight bearing on the painful hip. With the patient lying supine, passive rotation at the hip joint is both restricted and painful. Passive flexion of the contralateral hip results in flexion on the affected side as the pelvis tilts, due to loss of full joint mobility. On occasion, following a fall, an impacted fracture produces the same clinical picture and is diagnosed by X ray. Fear of hip fracture because of a previous fracture or its occurrence in a friend or relative often contributes to limitation of mobility and fear of falling in elderly patients. The fear is not irrational; a quarter of a million hip fractures occur in United States every year, with a mortality rate in the first year after hip fracture of 12–29%.

Pain in sciatic distribution is sometimes a symptom of trochanteric bursitis. The patient complains not only of sciatic pain but severe pain on changing from a sitting to an erect posture and cannot lie on the affected side. Exquisite point tenderness over the greater trochanter makes the diagnosis. At times, the tenderness extends a few inches distally down the lateral aspect of thigh, suggesting a more diffuse fasciitis. Local steroid injections are usually effective. Local tenderness at the anterior superior iliac spine associated with a patch of decreased sensitivity of varying size over the lateral thigh makes the diagnosis of meralgia paresthetica, and a local injection of steroid and local anesthetic are of symptomatic value. Often, meralgia and trochanteric bursitis coincide.

THE LUMBAR SPINE

Low-back pain with or without root pain is said to affect 90% of the population at some time and may affect walking. A good approach to back pain is to consider the differential diagnosis in terms of pain sensitive structures of the back. These are the bones, joints, discs, nerve roots, and paraspinal muscles. A physical examination and appropriate further imaging studies make the diagnosis.

Osteoporosis

Although routine X rays are relatively insensitive to detecting significant bone loss, 30% of elderly women and 20% of elderly men have osteoporosis, and about one third of women older than 65 have suffered either a vertebral or hip fracture related to osteoporosis. By the age of 80, half the female population will have evidence of vertebral fractures and close to 30% of women will have suffered a hip fracture. Vertebral fractures may be asymptomatic, producing only loss of height and kyphosis if the thoracic spine is involved but can be exquisitely painful, and the pain is aggravated by movement. Tenderness of the vertebral spines to light percussion is suggestive of osteoporosis, but metastatic deposits must be considered in the differential diagnosis. Extensive imaging may be necessary to make the diagnosis.

Claudication

Unilateral or bilateral sciatic pain or numbness in sciatic distribution precipitated by walking a set distance suggests the diagnosis of spinal neurogenic claudication. The neurologic examination at rest may be entirely normal, but after exercise, an ankle jerk may temporarily disappear, slight weakness may be found, or radicular sensory loss may make a transient appearance. In patients with neurogenic claudication, the peripheral pulses are normal. In elderly patients, the likely pathology is degenerative osteoarthritis of the lumbar spine with acquired spinal stenosis. On rare occasions, true vascular claudication of the cauda equina presents in exactly the same way, and imaging fails to demonstrate spinal stenosis or lumbar disc disease. These patients have stenosis of the internal iliac or ileohypogastric vessels, which supply the cauda. Pain in the legs with walking may be due to true claudication of the lower limbs—these patients will have absent pedal pulses, elevation pallor, dependency rubor, and delayed venous filling.

Lumbar Disc Degeneration

The elderly population is prone to lumbar disc degeneration and may present with severe sciatic pain and low-back pain sufficient to interfere with ambulation. Examination in these patients almost always reveals root dysfunction. Because the L4 and L5 discs are most commonly affected, there is likely to be atrophy and weakness of extensor digitorum brevis on the dorsal aspect of the foot, together with weakness of toe extension, hamstring, and thigh abduction. Some sensory loss may be found over the anterolateral leg or dorsal aspect of the foot. If the S1 root is involved, there will be weakness of toe flexion, occasionally of ankle flexion, and frequently an absent Achilles reflex. Sensory loss, if present, involves the lateral aspect of the foot.

High lumbar radiculopathy may result in the syndrome of anterior thigh pain and weakness of quadriceps. These patients have difficulty locking the knee when taking weight and may fall because the knee gives way.

Diabetic amyotrophy presents with a similar clinical picture, and differentiation of lumbar plexopathy or femoral neuritis from a radiculopathy may be difficult. If all muscles supplied by the L2–L3 roots are weak, radiculopathy is likely; but if the myotome is only partially affected, the site of the lesion is likely to be more distal than the root. Thus, a combination of weakness of hip flexion, thigh abduction, and knee extension is likely to be radicular, whereas if any two of three muscles are weak but the third remains strong, a plexopathy is likely. Single muscle weakness suggests dysfunction of the nerve supplying that muscle.

While lower lumbar root dysfunction and pain is overwhelmingly mechanical in origin and due to disc degeneration, in the mix will be some patients with nondiscogenic lesions. Bearing this in mind, if the symptoms and signs are bilateral or if they fail to resolve over 2–3 weeks, imaging of the lumbar spine is indicated. Imaging is also indicated if there are bladder symptoms, which might suggest cauda equina compression.

THE CARDIORESPIRATORY SYSTEM

Many patients with cardiorespiratory insufficiency complain simply of being exhausted; they describe loss of energy for walking. More specifically, a history of tightness in the chest or frank chest pain while walking strongly suggests the diagnosis of coronary artery disease. Dyspnea of effort may suggest either cardiac or pulmonary insufficiency. On occasion, postural hypotension of the central type may result in a fall in blood pressure only after being upright for a few minutes rather than immediately on standing, and the resultant disequilibrium may not at first glance be linked to the upright posture. Occasionally, an arrhythmia comes on while walking and is the cause of vertigo and imbalance. Cardiac monitoring should be considered in patients with intermittent symptoms with no obvious precipitating cause or if palpitations are prominent.

DRUGS

A careful review of medication that the patient is taking is essential. Many drugs cause postural hypotension, and sedatives and hypnotics are associated with an increased prevalence of falls. Overdoses of anticonvulsants produce ataxia, and vertigo can be caused by aminoglycoside antibiotics.

It is worth keeping in mind a list of those drugs associated with postural hypotension, because they are frequently prescribed and not well tolerated by the elderly. The drugs include diuretics and hypotensive agents, psychotropic drugs such as antidepressants and phenothiazines, and cardiac drugs such as nitrates, procainamide, and beta-blockers.

VISION

The movement of the body in space generates a continuously changing optic flow field that is used to assess the direction and speed of movement and utilized in a predictive mode so that locomotion is adapted to uneven terrain or to avoid obstacles. The visual system and vigilance, or attention, are the keys to the early detection of potential balance threats. Older adults have longer latencies for visual monitoring, and a longer time is required to implement gait modifications and adjust step length in response to a visual cue. Although the precise mechanisms have yet to be worked out, feed-forward information from the visual signal is relayed via visual and association cortices to the basal ganglia and cerebellum and thence to the thalamus and motor cortex. Feed-forward networks interact with feedback information from the peripheral and interneuronal networks in the spinal cord that make up the central pattern generator, and information is relayed to cerebellum and thalamus and thence to the motor cortex.

Visual information is important for normal locomotion in environments where the orientation of the world has to be continuously updated, distances toward various targets have to be continuously upgraded, locomotion has to be maintained in a certain direction or at a certain velocity, and obstacles have to be avoided. It is possible for a normal subject to walk for a certain distance with the eyes closed as long as they are opened periodically to allow reassessment of the environment and the position relative to it. However, the distance that can be reliably covered with the eyes closed is limited by the space (5 m) and the time (8 sec) of retention of the visual information.

It is impossible to change the direction of locomotion (30 or 60° change either way) within a one-step cycle if the visual cue to change direction is given after the foot has touched the ground. However, it is possible to stop or to change the step length and step height to accommodate an obstacle when the visual cue is given within the same step cycle. It is interesting to note that the long cane used by blind people is approximately one step length ahead so that there would be just enough time to correct the course of locomotion when detecting an obstacle with such an instrument.

Given the preceding, it is easy to understand the role of failing vision in gait disorders of the elderly. Progressive loss of vision leads to an uncertain, tentative gait and is frequently part of a multifactorial gait failure. The addition of visual failure to another cause of gait disorder is more than additive. In particular, in patients with posterior column dysfunction and loss of position sense, loss of visual clues can be devastating. Furthermore, many of the causes of visual failure are treatable; and evaluation of the patient with failing gait should include tests of visual acuity, visual fields, and inspection of the optic fundi at the bedside. Where appropriate, an ophthalmologic consultation and treatment of cataracts or glaucoma can be crucial in the management of patients with gait disorders.

SUGGESTED READING

Cavanagh PR, Rodgers MM, Iiboshi A. Pressure distribution under symptom-free feet during barefoot standing. Foot Ankle 1987;7:262.

Chan CW, Rudins A. Foot biomechanics during walking and running. Mayo Clin Proc 1994;69:448.

Cumming RG, Miller JP, Kelsey JL, et al. Medications and multiple falls in elderly people: the St. Louis OASIS study. Age Ageing 1991;20:455.

Drew T, Jiang W, Kably B, Lavoie S. The role of the motor cortex in the control of the visually triggered gait modifications. Can J Physiol Pharmacol 1996;74:426.

Gerster JC. Plantar fasciitis and Achilles tendinitis among 150 cases of seronegative spondylarthritis. Rheum Rehabil 1980;19:218.

Grundy M, Tosh PA, McLeish RD, Smidt L. An investigation of the centers of pressure under the foot while walking. J Bone Joint Surg 1975;57B:98.

Gurwitz JH, Soumeri SB, Avorn J. Improving medication prescribing and utilization in the nursing home. J Am Geriatr Soc 1990;38:542.

Hutton WC, Dhanendran M. The mechanics of normal and hallux valgus feet—a quantitative study. Clin Orthop Rel Res 1981;157:7.

Lord SR, Clark RD, Webster IW. Visual acuity and contrast sensitivity in relation to falls in an elderly population. Age Ageing 1991;20:175.

MacDonald J. Falls in the elderly: the role of drugs in the elderly. Clin Geriatr Med 1985;1:621.

Mann RA, Mizel MS. Monoarticular nontraumatic synovitis of the metatarsophalangeal joint: a new diagnosis? Foot Ankle 1985;6:18.

Mizel MS. Physical examination of the foot. Video J Orthop 1992;7(6).

Ray WA, Griffin MR. Prescribed medications, falling, and fall-related injuries. In Weindruch R, Ory M (eds), Frailty Reconsidered: Reducing Frailty and Fall-Related Injuries in the Elderly. Springfield, IL: Charles C Thomas, 1991:76.

Rossignol S. Visuomotor regulation of locomotion. Can J Physiol Pharmacol 1996;74:418.

Snow RE, Williams KR, Holmes GB. The effects of wearing high-heeled shoes on pedal pressures in women. Foot Ankle 1992;13:85.

Steiger P, Cummings SR, Black DM, et al. Age-related decrements in bone mineral density in women over 65. J Bone Miner Res 1992;7:625.

Trepman E, Yeo S-J. Nonoperative treatment of metatarsophalangeal joint synovitis. Foot Ankle Int 1995; 16:771.

Wapner KL, Sharkey PF. The use of night splints treatment of recalcitrant plantar fasciitis. Foot Ankle 1991;12:135.

Falls in the Elderly

Falls have been defined as "events which lead to the conscious subject coming to rest inadvertently on the ground." By definition, this excludes episodes of loss of consciousness, but for purposes of discussion in this chapter, we include those falls associated with loss of consciousness, and the first branch on the decision tree is to separate falls without loss of consciousness from those in which consciousness is impaired.

INCIDENCE

The problem of falls in the elderly is significant (Table 10-1). According to the National Safety Council, among persons aged 65 years and over, falls were

Table 10-1. Falls in the elderly

Falling with loss of consciousness
    Syncope
        Arrhythmia
        Aortic stenosis
        Myocardial infarction
        Carotid sinus sensitivity
        Orthostatic hypotension
    Seizure
    Generalized
    Partial

Falling with no loss of consciousness
    Drop attacks
    Vestibular dysfunction
    Drug-related causes
    Orthostatic hypotension
    Confusional states due to acute systemic infection or
      organ dysfunction
    Cardiac pathology, arrhythmia, and carotid sinus
      sensitivity
    Orthopedic problems
    Neurologic causes such as stroke, extrapyramidal
      disease, spinal cord or root dysfunction, loss of
      proprioception, cerebellar ataxia, frontal gait disor-
      der, and progressive space-taking pathology within
      the skull
    Environmental hazards

the leading cause of death in 1987 and accounted for 33% of the death total for this age group. Accidents are the fifth leading cause of death in people aged 65 years and older and falls account for two thirds of those accidental deaths. Of deaths from falls in the United States, over 70% occurred in the 11% of the population over age 65, and with the baby boomers reaching maturity, these numbers are expected to increase.

In a year, 30% of those over 65 years and about 50% of those over 80 years will experience at least one fall, and it is estimated that 6–10% of falls in the elderly result in significant injury. Of those living at home who fall, about 1 in 40 will be hospitalized, and of those admitted to a hospital after a fall, only about half will be alive 1 year later. Among elderly people in institutions, 10–25% will have a serious fall each year.

Of elderly patients who fall, 50% are able to get up, most of these are not seriously injured. Inability to get up is a poor prognostic sign, associated with features suggestive of physical frailty, age 80 or older, weakness, poor balance, arthritis, and dependency in activities of daily living. Of those who fall, subsequent limitation of activity occurs in about 40%, whether due to physical impairment from injury or fear of future falls.

The problem in the elderly achieves greater magnitude not simply because of the frequency of falls. Young children and athletes have a higher incidence of falls, yet are not prone to severe injury. The frail elderly population with osteoporosis, slower protective reflexes, and normal age-related gait changes are more likely to sustain a serious injury.

A fracture is the most common injury, and the hip is the most common fracture to result in acute hospitalization. Of hip fractures, 84% occur in persons 65 years of age or older. Approximately 40% of older people with hip fractures die within 6 months of injury.

CAUSES

In considering the causes of falls in the elderly, one should review both environmental hazards and medical problems of the patients who fall. About 55% of falls are related to medically diagnosed conditions, and 37% are related to environmental hazards. Most falls occur during routine activities at home, including walking or going up or down steps, and about half of all falls can be classified as accidental and associated with an environmental hazard.

Poor lighting, inadequate stair railings, slippery flooring or bathtub, frayed carpets, and unstable furniture should be specifically looked for during home visits; these are amenable to manipulation. On patient examination, particular attention should be directed toward the possibility of impaired vision or hearing, a review of medications, and neurological disability. Frequently, multifactorial risk factors are found, and modification of at least some will reduce the risk of future falls.

FALLS WITH LOSS OF CONSCIOUSNESS

The establishment of loss of consciousness is history dependent, but it is often difficult to be sure. The patient often has a hard time describing the fall, and it is much easier to make a diagnosis if there is a witness. A good question to ask is, "Do you remember hitting the ground?"

Syncope

Palpitations, lightheadedness, and history of sweating before the episode suggest syncope. A witness account of color change is helpful, as is a history of cough, micturition, or extreme emotional distress immediately prior to the incident. Patients who faint, usually rapidly regain consciousness once they are horizontal, so that a history of prolonged loss of consciousness is against the diagnosis of syncope. On the other hand, some patients who faint have few myoclonic jerks before regaining consciousness as part of the syncopal episode, and a history of jerky movements of the limbs or body does not exclude the diagnosis of syncope.

Syncope implies transient cerebral hypoperfusion, yet no single cause can be established in up to 50% of patients. The most frequent single disorders implicated in syncope are myocardial infarction, aortic stenosis, and volume depletion. Occasional patients have carotid sinus sensitivity, where gentle massage of the carotid bifurcation in the neck with electrocardiogram (EKG) control precipitates bradycardia. If 5 seconds of massage produces >50% reduction in heart rate or a long pause of more than 2 seconds, this is diagnostic.

If there are no obvious precipitating causes, such as fainting on assuming the erect posture to suggest postural hypotension or a significant history of Valsalva-like maneuvers, a search for arrhythmia is warranted. A routine resting EKG is insufficient and will miss the majority of arrhythmias. If the elderly, even with no history of heart disease, are monitored, a multitude of abnormalities are often found, and cardiac arrhythmias detected by Holter monitoring can be implicated as a cause of falls associated with symptoms of dizziness, syncope, and drop attacks, although there is considerable overlap with normals. High-grade ventricular ectopy, sustained supraventricular tachycardias, and severe brady-arrhythmias should be treated appropriately.

Seizure

A witness history of tonic-clonic convulsions in all four extremities with tongue biting and urinary incontinence followed by a minute or so of unconsciousness and then postictal confusion is diagnostic of a grand mal seizure.

Some patients may be able to describe an aura preceding the seizure. The aura in partial epilepsy depends on the site of initial ictal discharge, and secondary generalization results in loss of consciousness. If the focal site is in the motor strip, there is a classical Jacksonian seizure with focal clonic movements of the hand or fingers that spread rapidly to proximal muscles and face and ultimately to the whole body, with loss of consciousness. The same principle holds for sensory seizures, where there is a dramatic rapid march over seconds with paresthesiae spreading up or down a limb or from limb to limb or face. Seizures arising in the frontal lobes may present with a drop attack, and seizures arising in the occipital lobes may present with unformed visual hallucinations. Seizures arising in mesial temporal areas present with hallucinations of taste, smell, or vision. At times, the hallucinations take the form of psychic manifestations, such as depersonalization or derealization.

An electroencephalogram (EEG) may demonstrate focal slowing or spike activity to support the notion of a partial seizure, but the diagnosis of seizure is essentially clinical, made at the bedside based on data acquired from the patient and witnesses. When the bedside diagnosis is unclear, the EEG will help, particularly if spike activity is seen.

FALLS WITH NO LOSS OF CONSCIOUSNESS

Falls in the elderly are often of multifactorial origin. Evaluation demands a painstaking and thorough assessment, and one should consider neurologic, nonneurologic, and environmentally triggered problems.

Although the patient occasionally pinpoints the cause, the history, often taken some time after the incident, may be unhelpful—"I lost my balance," "my legs gave way," or "I just fell." It is important to ferret out the exact circumstances of the fall and determine what medication the patient takes.

Drop Attacks

A drop attack is a fall due to sudden loss of tone or power in the legs with no loss of consciousness. The pathophysiology of true drop attacks, which are relatively rare, is unknown. They seem to be more frequent in elderly women, and vertebrobasilar insufficiency is an often quoted but unproven cause. In the differential diagnosis, one should consider cataplexy, a myoclonic jerk, or a frontal seizure.

Vestibular Dysfunction

True rotary vertigo is an uncommon cause of falling, but nonspecific dizziness, disequilibrium, and general unsteadiness are common in elderly patients and may precipitate a fall. Testing for vestibular dysfunction is described in Chapter 4. Cervical vertigo is discussed in Chapter 11. Patients with dizziness and disequilibrium are often anxious, depressed, and afraid of falling.

Drugs

A detailed drug history is mandatory. Diuretics may be implicated in hypovolemia, and antihypertensives may be the cause of hypotension. Tranquilizers, antidepressants, and sedatives substantially increase the risk of falls and hip fractures. Alcohol should not be forgotten.

Orthostatic Hypotension

The blood pressure should be measured with the patient supine and standing. Because of the possibility of delayed postural hypotension, the patient should be kept standing for 3 or 4 minutes and the systolic blood pressure measured again; a postural drop in systolic pressure of more than 20 points is significant.

A compensatory tachycardia suggests the diagnosis of hypovolemia. Lack of a compensatory tachycardia in hypovolemic patients suggests either that the cardiac response is blocked by drugs or that there is a primary cardiac disease. Postprandial orthostatic hypotension should be considered in the differential diagnosis of patients who "eat and sink."

Neurogenic autonomic failure may be central or peripheral in origin. In peripheral dysfunction, the fall in blood pressure frequently is immediate; and in central dysfunction, it may be delayed. Many patients with Parkinson's disease have postural hypotension, but if the autonomic dysfunction is dominant, "systems degeneration" should be considered.

Confusional State

This cause of falling and gait disorder is often overlooked. *Confusion* is defined as the inability to carry out a coherent stream of thought or action. The majority of elderly patients who are confused have no primary brain dysfunction to cause confusion but, by virtue of a mild or moderate degenerative disease or dementia, are exceptionally vulnerable to the effects of exogenous or endogenous toxins of all sorts. Usually organ failure, sepsis, or exogenous toxin is the cause.

The patient may fall either because of asterixis or myoclonus affecting the legs or simply because of a central disequilibrium. A fall can herald the onset of a variety of acute illnesses ("premonitoring falls"). Fever, tachypnea, tachycardia, and hypotension indicate sepsis, myocardial infarction, pulmonary embolus, or GI bleeding as possible systemic illnesses.

Cardiac Pathology

The cardiac mechanisms of syncope can cause falls with no frank loss of consciousness, and a cardiac workup may be indicated if no other obvious cause is found.

Neurologic Causes of Falling

Any cause of gait disorder could be a cause of falling. The approach should be simple and basic: Is there weakness, impaired vision, ataxia, extrapyramidal disease, deafferentation, or frontal dysfunction? The neurologic examination will give the answer, and further studies are dictated by the physical examination.

Orthopedic Problems

Orthopedic problems may be as mundane as a local cause for pain in the foot causing the patient to stumble and fall or as complicated as hip arthritis.

Attention to the feet is important: calluses, bunions, toe deformities, and ill-fitting shoes may cause pain and instability. If there is pain in the foot on taking weight, an interdigital neuroma, plantar fasciitis, or even a calcaneal spur should be considered. Side-to-side compression of the metatarsal heads with local tenderness when pressure is applied from the plantar aspect of the foot suggests Morton's metatarsalgia due to an interdigital neuroma. Local tenderness in the sole of the foot suggests plantar fasciitis, and local tenderness at the medial anterior aspect of the calcaneum suggests a spur. More severe orthopedic problems may be revealed by limitation of movement, pain, or deformity of the knees, hips, and back. Lumbar root compression due to disc or spur, apart from causing pain in the back and sciatica, may cause weakness of toe or foot extension so that the patient is liable to trip and fall as the toes catch on thick rugs or minor protuberances on the ground.

SUMMARY

Falls may or may not be associated with loss of consciousness. If there is loss of consciousness, consider syncope or seizure. If there is no loss of consciousness, the diagnosis of the cause is based on assessment of environmental hazards and patient pathology. The cause is often multifactorial and treatment is diagnosis driven.

SUGGESTED READING

Cummings RG, Miller PJ, Kelsy JL, et al. Medications and multiple falls in elderly people: the St. Louis OASIS study. Age and Ageing 1991;20:455.

Kapoor WN. Syncope in older persons. J Am Geriatr Soc 1994;42:426.

Lipsitz LA, Jonsson PV, Kelley MM, Koestner JS. Causes and correlates of recurrent falls in ambulatory frail elderly. J Gerontol 1991;46:M114.

Lipsitz LA, Nyquist RP, Wei JY. Postprandial reduction in blood pressure in the elderly. N Engl J Med 1983; 309:81.

Nevitt MC, Cummings SR, Kidd S, Black D. Risk factors for recurrent nonsyncopal falls. JAMA 1989;261: 2663.

Rubenstein LR, Robbins AS, Schulman BL, et al. Falls and instability in the elderly. J Am Geriatr Soc 1988;36: 266.

Sattin RW, Lambert Huber DA, DeVito CA, et al. The incidence of fall injury events among the elderly in a defined population. Am J Epidemiol 1990;131: 1028.

Tideiksaar R. Falls in the elderly. Bull NY Acad Med 1988;64:145.

Tinetti ME, Speechley M, Ginter SF. Risk factors for falls among elderly persons living in the community. N Engl J Med 1988;19:1701.

Walker JE, Howland J. Falls and fear of falling among elderly persons living in the community: occupational therapy interventions. Am J Occup Ther 1991;45:119.

Cervical Spondylosis

Myelopathy caused by cervical spondylosis with cervical stenosis is a frequent cause of gait disorders in the elderly. In one study of patients with gait disorder, myelopathy was the cause in 16.7% of the patients. Because of its frequency, the clinical syndrome merits a specific chapter.

The term *cervical spondylosis* is used to describe a degenerative disorder of the cervical spine characterized by disc softening, desiccation, and shrinking with secondary osteophyte formation, spurring, and ridging and overgrowth of the facet joints. Apart from pain and stiffness in the neck and headache, the more significant clinical symptoms and signs are related to nerve root and spinal cord compression. Cervical cord dysfunction has an impact on gait. As always, the diagnosis is made by careful clinical examination, which invariably reveals the relevant clinical signs.

Cervical spondylosis is common; it is estimated that 50% of people older than 50 years and 75% of people older than 65 years have typical radiological changes of cervical spondylosis. Furthermore, 40% of people older than 50 years have some limitation of neck movement, and 60% have some neurological abnormality if examined carefully. Little correlation exists between the degree of anatomical abnormality and the clinical presentation, and the natural history and treatment options have never been prospectively studied.

SPINAL STENOSIS

A congenitally narrowed spinal canal predisposes to myelopathy. Therefore, even exuberant osteophytes in the setting of a wide canal do not affect the cervical cord, whereas relatively mild spurring, ridging, or hypertrophy of the posterior ligamentum flavum in the presence of a narrow canal may cause cord compression, especially in the extremes of neck flexion or extension. Massive osteophytes and ligamentous hypertrophy occasionally compress the cord even in the absence of congenital spinal stenosis.

The canal diameter is easily measured on lateral radiographs, and a posterior-anterior diameter of less than 14 mm renders the cord vulnerable to compression in cervical spondylosis. The spinal dimensions in patients with spondylotic myelopathy range from 7 to 17 mm. With neck extension, there is bulging of the ligamentum flavum, which causes a pincer-like effect from behind; and with neck flexion, the cord rides forward, and impacts on posteriorly projecting osteophytes and ridges. The mechanics may be further disrupted by loose ligaments, which allow for subluxation of the cervical spine in flexion/extension movements. Patients with minor cord compression are at risk to develop severe myelopathy in the event of trauma, particularly in motor vehicle accidents, where flexion extension injuries are common, and sometimes at intubation for anesthesia for surgical procedures, where hyperextension of the neck is favored by the anesthesiologist.

The precise pathogenesis of myelopathy in cervical stenosis is not entirely clear. If simple cord compression were the prime pathophysiology, adequate surgical decompression should arrest or cure the condition. A small percentage of patients, however, continue to deteriorate despite cord decompression. Various explanations other than simple compression have been offered. These include edema and demyelination as well as vascular compromise of the cord. On occasion magnetic resonance imaging will demonstrate T2 bright areas within the cord at the level of spurring. If these resolve with treatment, the only explanation is edema; if they persist, then it is likely that permanent gliosis has ensued. Demyelination has been observed at autopsy, but no pathology in the anterior spinal artery has ever been demonstrated. Blood flow in radicular feeding vessels, however, could be compromised by root fibrosis.

With flexion and extension of the neck, the cord moves up and down the canal and may rub against osteophytes anteriorly and the ligamentum flavum posteriorly. Use of a cervical collar eliminates or restricts flexion/extension movements and frequently results in clinical improvement of myelopathy.

The spinothalamic and posterior column tract anatomy has been likened to an onion peel, arranged in somatotopic fashion—in the spinothalamic tract, the most peripheral parts of the tract carry sensation from sacral dermatomes; and in orderly fashion from the outer part of the tract to the inner parts, there follows foot, leg, trunk, and arm areas. In the posterior columns, the more lateral parts of the tract carry sensation from the arms; and the central part of the tract carries sensation from the feet. When the cervical cord is compressed, dysfunction can be patchy, progressive, or both, resulting in a wide variation of sensory loss. Sparing of pinprick sensation around the anus (sacral sparing) suggests dysfunction in the central part of cord with preservation of the more peripheral parts, but does not help in distinguishing primary pathology within the cord itself from extrinsic cord compression as in cervical spondylosis.

Wasting and weakness of the hypothenar muscles and pinprick sensory loss over the hypothenar eminence is commonly seen, suggesting low cervical radiculopathy. But the maximal pathology in cervical spondylosis is usually at around the C5–C6 and C6–C7 levels. It has been suggested that, in spinal stenosis, there may be obstruction to normal venous drainage, which is thought to be craniad, with maximal venous distention and stagnant anoxia maximal at the C8–T1 level to explain the signs. This pseudoulnar syndrome is sometimes seen with high cord compression, even at the level of the foramen magnum.

CLINICAL PRESENTATION

Symptoms

Patients with gait disorder due to cervical spondylosis may or may not have symptoms related to the neck, but a history of stiff neck, muscle-contraction-type headache, previous automobile accident or other trauma, and occasionally a Lhermitte symptom help with localization. Brachialgia may point the way.

Almost never can the patient pinpoint the cause of the gait disorder—the complaint is simply "I can't walk" or "I keep falling," occasionally, "it's my legs." Hip flexor weakness may cause difficulty climbing stairs, toe extensor weakness may cause the toes to catch on steps, ground irregularities, or thick rugs resulting in tripping. Spasticity results in scuffing of the feet, and loss of proprioception occasionally result in the complaint that the patient has more difficulty with walking in the dark and falls at night.

Bladder symptoms may be the clue to cervical myelopathy but are not universal. The upper motor neuron bladder is small and spastic, and this results in frequency, urgency, and urgency incontinence. Spinal cord dysfunction at a lower level can result in bladder dyssynergia; the detrusor contracts on a closed sphincter and the patient experiences the usual, often urgent, desire to urinate but cannot initiate micturation.

Signs

Localization of the segmental level of cord pathology depends on the demonstration of root signs.

These may include myotomal wasting or weakness, a dropped tendon reflex, or dermatomal sensory loss. Occasionally, widespread fasciculations in the upper limbs are due to cervical radiculopathy.

Myelopathic signs of varying degree are to be found in the lower limbs but are not strictly correlated with the pathology demonstrated on imaging studies.

Any combination of the following physical signs may be found, or they may exist in isolation:

- *Spasticity* alone results in a narrow-based gait with the thighs adducted and the tendency to catch the toes so that a scraping sound can be heard with each step. On the couch, the examiner rotates the relaxed leg from side to side to find that the feet are held fairly rigid at the ankles. Frank clasp knife rigidity may be present at the knees, and clonus may present at the ankles.
- Upper motor neuron *weakness* in the lower limbs is seen in a specific pattern. There is weakness solely or mainly in hip flexors, ankle and toe dorsiflexors, hamstrings, and thigh abductors.
- The knee and ankle *tendon reflexes* are likely increased, but the plantar responses are variable. *Extensor plantar responses* indicate pyramidal tract dysfunction, but flexor plantar responses do not exclude cervical myelopathy.

The significant sensory signs in patients with gait disorders due to cervical spondylosis are those relating to the posterior columns. *Position sense* may be defective when tested at the big toes; and in patients with more subtle dysfunction, the deficit will be found only in the little toes. Romberg's sign is positive.

Cord dysfunction may also result in sensory loss in cape distribution in the upper limbs as the result of central cord dysfunction due to extrinsic cord compression, and spinothalamic tract dysfunction can result in variable areas of sensory loss on the trunk and lower limbs.

Management

The diagnosis of spondylotic myelopathy is made at the bedside, based on the finding of motor or sensory signs suggesting cord dysfunction in the setting of restricted and often painful neck movement. The diagnosis needs to be confirmed and other pathology excluded, so that the cervical spine needs to be imaged. Magnetic resonance imaging (MRI) is the modality of choice.

Because there are no prospective controlled trials of conservative versus surgical management of spondylotic myelopathy, the choice of treatment is, in large measure, one of judgment. The debate continues, with some protagonists favoring a conservative approach and others surgical decompression. Rowland reviewed the literature in 1992. Of 261 patients subjected to posterior cervical laminectomy, 60% improved, 34% were unchanged, and 6% were worse. Of 385 patients surgically treated by an anterior approach, 52% were better, 24% were unchanged, and 23% were worse after the operation. Of 136 patients treated conservatively without surgery, 44% improved, 33% were unchanged, and 23% deteriorated. The perioperative morbidity was generally in the range of 4–5%. No prospective controlled trial of conservative versus surgical treatment has ever been done.

Some studies suggest a better outcome with surgery in selected patients. More modern studies, admittedly retrospective, suggest that one might expect 50% of patients to return to full employment and another 30–40% return to light employment 2–3 months after surgery. Saunders reports an 89.7% success rate with corpectomy. Tarlov reports 56% improvement, 30% stabilization, and 10% worsening with posterior decompression, numbers not far removed from the Rowland review.

If myelopathy is present but the cord is not severely compressed, so that one can still see spinal fluid (white on T2) around the cord, a more conservative approach is suggested. If the cord is severely compressed and signs in the lower limbs are significant, a neurosurgical opinion is warranted. Significant sub-luxation on flexion/extension radiographs of the cervical spine may indicate surgical fusion. Because cervical spondylotic myelopathy is frequently a problem in the elderly, coexisting disease may contraindicate surgery despite severe pathology, but age itself is no contraindication to surgical treatment.

Conservative management implies the use of a cervical collar. The patient is instructed to wear the collar continually—that is, all day and all night for 3–4 weeks and then to continue to sleep in the collar for an indefinite period of time. These patients require careful monitoring and should be reexamined at regular intervals. Failure to respond or progression would suggest a reconsideration of the possibility of surgical intervention. For pain, analgesics and muscle relaxants, and in patients who have chronic pain, antidepressant therapy are all valuable adjuncts. Gentle physical therapy avoiding cervical manipulation and strenuous neck exercise is sometimes of symptomatic benefit.

Chiropractic manipulation is mentioned only to condemn it. Approximately 12 million Americans undergo spinal manipulation therapy every year; the only published randomized controlled trial of chiropractic manipulation did not demonstrate that the maneuver was significantly helpful. One review described 138 cases with serious complications, including posterior circulation stroke and even death. Cervical manipulation in patients with cord compression can aggravate the myelopathy.

In patients who are denied surgery because of comorbidity or lack of consent to a surgical approach, conservative treatment implies a survey of the home for risks of falling and the use of appropriate aids to facilitate activities of daily living.

Surgery in cervical spondylosis is generally reserved for fit patients with myelopathy. It is rarely beneficial in patients without clear-cut radiological evidence of cord compression, regardless of the clinical presentation. While the gold standard for diagnosis is MRI, occasionally computed tomography is helpful in delineating calcification in the anterior or posterior longitudinal ligaments. Lateral radiographs of the cervical spine with flexion and extension are important to exclude significant subluxation.

The aim of surgery is adequate decompression of the spinal cord and nerve roots in the cervical spine. Many surgeons favor anterior cervical decompression with fusion if there is cord compression at one or two levels—the spine is stabilized with an iliac crest strut graft. For more extensive pathology, a more radical approach is sometimes used, even to the extent of the anterior median corpectomy from C2 to C7 with stabilization of the spine using a cadaver fibula graft as a strut in the midline. With multilevel cord compression, a posterior cervical laminectomy with bilateral partial facetectomy and foramenotomy is less technically challenging and better tolerated. The exact approach should be the decision of the surgeon. It seems reasonable to suggest that the direction of approach should be the most direct and shortest route to the site of greatest cord compression. Certainly, there is no statistical evidence to support either the anterior or posterior approach, and the more radical procedures remain to be proven.

If surgery is contemplated, the complication rate should be discussed. Poor outcomes were reviewed by Clifton: In his study, the causes were wrong diagnosis (14.3%), spinal cord atrophy (26.8%), diffuse spinal stenosis (28.6%), and failure of decompression (57.1%). A bright spot on T2 magnetic resonance images is also a poor prognostic sign. The complications of anterior decompression and fusion include damage to the esophagus and recurrent laryngeal nerve, graft failure, and cord or root damage.

Given the absence of proof, it would seem acceptable to adopt a more conservative approach in patients with mild cord compression and relatively minor signs and a surgical approach if there is no response to neck immobilization. For patients with a more severe gait disorder, neurogenic bladder, and significant cord compression, a surgical approach seems more reasonable.

SUGGESTED READING

Adams CBT, Logue V. Studies in cervical spondylotic myelopathy. Brain 1971;94:557.

Adams CBT, Logue V. Studies in cervical spondylotic myelopathy II. Movement and contour of the spine in relation to the neural complications of cervical spondylosis. Brain 1971;94:569.

Bohlman HH, Emery SE. The pathophysiology of cervical spondylosis and myelopathy. Spine 1988;13:843.

Brain WR, Wilkinson M. Cervical Spondylosis and Other Disorders of the Cervical Spine. Philadelphia: Saunders, 1967.

Clifton AG, Stevens JM, Whitear P, Kendall BE. Identifiable cause for poor outcome in surgery for cervical spondylosis. Neuroradiology 1990;32:450.

Elsberg GA. The extradural ventral chondromas (ecchondroses), their favorite sites, the spinal cord and root symptoms they produce, and their surgical treatment. Bull Neurol Inst NY 1931;1:350.

Fairbank J. Trials and tribulations in cervical spondylosis. (editorial). Lancet 1998;352:1165.

Gooding MR, Wilson CB, Hoff J. Experimental cervical myelopathy: effects of ischemia and compression of the canine cervical cord. J Neurosurg 1975;43:9.

Nurick S. The natural history and results of surgical treatment of the spinal cord disorder associated with cervical spondylosis. Brain 1972;95:101.

Powell FC, Hanigan WC, Olivero WC. A risk/benefit analysis of spinal manipulation for relief of lumbar or cervical pain. Neurosurgery 1993;33:73.

Ronthal M. Neck Complaints. Boston: Butterworth–Heinemann, 2000.

Ronthal M, Rachlin JR. Cervical spondylosis. In Johnson RT, Griffin JW (eds), Current Therapy in Neurologic Disease, 5th ed. St. Louis: Mosby, 1997:76.

Rowland LP. Surgical treatment of cervical spondylotic myelopathy: time for a controlled trial. Neurology 1992;42:5.

Saunders RL. Anterior and middle column decompression. In Saunders RL, Bernini PM (eds), Cervical Spondylotic Myelopathy. Boston: Blackwell, 1992.

Snow RB, Weiner H. Cervical laminectomy and foramenotomy as surgical treatment of cervical spondylosis: a follow up study with analysis of failures. J Spinal Disord 1993;6:245; discussion:250.

Tarlov EC. Posterior column decompression in cervical spondylotic myelopathy. In Saunders RL, Bernini PM (eds), Cervical Spondylotic Myelopathy. Boston: Blackwell, 1992.

Wilkinson M. Cervical Spondylosis: Its Early Diagnosis and Treatment. Philadelphia: Saunders, 1971.

Index

Page references followed by "t" denote tables; "f" denote figures.